Sexually Transmitted Infections

Editor

SUSAN TUDDENHAM

MEDICAL CLINICS OF NORTH AMERICA

www.medical.theclinics.com

Consulting Editor
JACK ENDE

March 2024 • Volume 108 • Number 2

ELSEVIER

1600 John F. Kennedy Boulevard • Suite 1800 • Philadelphia, Pennsylvania, 19103-2899

http://www.theclinics.com

MEDICAL CLINICS OF NORTH AMERICA Volume 108, Number 2
March 2024 ISSN 0025-7125, ISBN-13: 978-0-443-12905-6

Editor: Taylor Hayes
Developmental Editor: Malvika Shah

Medical Clinics of North America (ISSN 0025-7125) is published bimonthly by Elsevier Inc., 360 Park Avenue South, New York, NY 10010-1710. Months of publication are January, March, May, July, September, and November. Business and editorial offices: 1600 John F. Kennedy Boulevard, Suite 1800, Philadelphia, PA 19103-2899. Periodicals postage paid at New York, NY, and additional mailing offices. Subscription prices are USD $336.00 per year (US individuals), $100.00 per year (US Students), $433.00 per year (Canadian individuals), $200.00 per year for (foreign students), $100.00 per year for (Canadian students), $479.00 per year (foreign individuals). For institutional access pricing please contact Customer Service via the contact information below. To receive student/resident rate, orders must be accompanied by name of affiliated institution, date of term, and the signature of program/residency coordinator on institution letterhead. Orders will be billed at individual rate until proof of status is received. Foreign air speed delivery is included in all Clinics' subscription prices. All prices are subject to change without notice. **POSTMASTER:** Send address changes to *Medical Clinics of North America*, Elsevier Health Sciences Division, Subscription Customer Service, 3251 Riverport Lane, Maryland Heights, MO 63043. **Customer Service: Telephone: 1-800-654-2452** (U.S. and Canada); **1-314-447-8871** (outside U.S. and Canada). **Fax: 314-447-8029. E-mail: journalscustomerserviceusa@elsevier.com** (for print support); **journalsonlinesupport-usa@elsevier.com** (for online support).

Reprints. For copies of 100 or more of articles in this publication, please contact the Commercial Reprints Department, Elsevier Inc., 360 Park Avenue South, New York, NY 10010-1710. Tel.: 212-633-3874; Fax: 212-633-3820; E-mail: reprints@elsevier.com.

Medical Clinics of North America is also published in Spanish by McGraw-Hill Interamericana Editores S. A., P.O. Box 5-237, 06500 Mexico, D.F., Mexico.

Medical Clinics of North America is covered in *MEDLINE/PubMed (Index Medicus), Current Contents, ASCA, Excerpta Medica, Science Citation Index, and ISI/BIOMED.*

PROGRAM OBJECTIVE

The goal of the *Medical Clinics of North America* is to keep practicing physicians up to date with current clinical practice by providing timely articles reviewing the state of the art in patient care.

TARGET AUDIENCE

All practicing physicians and other healthcare professionals.

LEARNING OBJECTIVES

Upon completion of this activity, participants will be able to:

1. Review strategies to promote sex-positive healthcare practice in clinical settings and beyond.
2. Explain the importance of taking a patient's sexual health history with sensitivity, inclusivity, and a trauma-informed perspective.
3. Discuss challenges primary care clinicians face associated with the management of common sexually transmitted infections (STIs).

ACCREDITATION

The Elsevier Office of Continuing Medical Education (EOCME) is accredited by the Accreditation Council for Continuing Medical Education (ACCME) to provide continuing medical education for physicians.

The EOCME designates this journal-based CME activity for a maximum of 12 *AMA PRA Category 1 Credit*(s)™. Physicians should claim only the credit commensurate with the extent of their participation in the activity.

All other healthcare professionals requesting continuing education credit for this enduring material will be issued a certificate of participation.

DISCLOSURE OF CONFLICTS OF INTEREST

The EOCME assesses conflict of interest with its instructors, faculty, planners, and other individuals who are in a position to control the content of CME activities. All relevant conflicts of interest that are identified are thoroughly vetted by EOCME for fair balance, scientific objectivity, and patient care recommendations. EOCME is committed to providing its learners with CME activities that promote improvements or quality in healthcare and not a specific proprietary business or a commercial interest.

The planning committee, staff, authors, and editors listed below have identified no financial relationships or relationships to products or devices they or their spouse/life partner have with commercial interest related to the content of this CME activity:

Luis F. Barroso, II, MD; Teresa A. Batteiger, MD, MS; Chase A. Cannon, MD, MPH; Joseph Cherabie, MD, MSc; Elizabeth A. Gilliams, MD, MSc; Shauna Gunaratne, MD, MPH, DTM&H; Matthew M. Hamill, MBChB, PhD; Donald Hong, MD; Michelle Littlejohn; Zachary Lorenz, MD; Stephanie E. McLaughlin, MD, MPH; Jacob McLean, DO; Masayo Nishiyama, RN, DNP; Oluyomi Obafemi, MD MPH; Merlin Packiam; Laura A.S. Quilter, MD, MPH; Asa Radix, MD, PhD, MPH, FACP; Meena Ramchandani, MD, MPH; Cornelis A. Rietmeijer, MD, PhD; Sarah Rowan, MD; Sancta B. St. Cyr, MD, MPH; Golsa M. Yazdy, MD; Jason Zucker, MD, MS

The planning committee, staff, authors, and editors listed below have identified financial relationships or relationships to products or devices they or their spouse/life partner have with commercial interest related to the content of this CME activity:

Kevin L. Ard, MD, MPH: Researcher: Binx Health, Inc.

Lindley A. Barbee, MD, MPH: Researcher: Hologic, Inc., Nabriva Therapeutics plc, SpeeDx Pty. Ltd.

Keosha T. Bond, EdD, MPH, CHES: Researcher: Gilead Sciences, Inc.

A.C. Demidont, MD: Employee: Gilead Sciences, Inc.

Andrew MacDonald-Ly, PharmD, AAHIVP: Employee: Gilead Sciences, Inc.

Kenneth H. Mayer, MD: Researcher: Gilead Sciences, Inc, Merck, Inc, ViiV Healthcare; Advisor: Gilead Sciences, Inc, Pfizer.

Candice J. McNeil, MD, MPH: Researcher: GlaxoSmithKline, BD, Cepheid, Gilead Sciences, Inc., Hologic, Inc.; Advisor: Tallo Biomedical.

Caroline Mitchell, MD, MPH: Consultant: Ferring Pharmaceuticals, Scynexis, Inc.; Researcher: Scynexis, Inc.

Hilary E. Reno, MD, PhD: Researcher: Hologic, Inc.

Jack D. Sobel, MD: Consultant: Scynexis, Inc., Mycovia Pharmaceuticals, Inc.

Susan Tuddenham, MD, MPH: Consultant: BioFire Diagnostics, F. Hoffmann-La Roche Ltd, Luca Biologics, Inc.; Speaker: F. Hoffmann-La Roche Ltd; Researcher: Hologic, Inc.

Karen Wendel, MD: Researcher: Hologic, Inc.

Kimberly Workowski, MD: Researcher: AbbVie, Inc., Gilead Sciences, Inc.

UNAPPROVED/OFF-LABEL USE DISCLOSURE

The EOCME requires CME faculty to disclose to the participants;

1. When products or procedures being discussed are off-label, unlabelled, experimental, and/or investigational (not US Food and Drug Administration [FDA] approved); and
2. Any limitations on the information presented, such as data that are preliminary or that represent ongoing research, interim analyses, and/or unsupported opinions. Faculty may discuss information about pharmaceutical agents that is outside of FDA-approved labelling. This information is intended solely for CME and is not intended to promote off-label use of these medications. If you have any questions, contact the medical affairs department of the manufacturer for the most recent prescribing information.

TO ENROLL

To enroll in the *Medical Clinics of North America* Continuing Medical Education program, call customer service at 1-800-654-2452 or sign up online at http://www.theclinics.com/home/cme. The CME program is available to subscribers for an additional annual fee of USD 319.00.

METHOD OF PARTICIPATION

In order to claim credit, participants must complete the following;

1. Complete enrolment as indicated above.
2. Read the activity.
3. Complete the CME Test and Evaluation. Participants must achieve a score of 70% on the test. All CME Tests and Evaluations must be completed online.

CME INQUIRIES/SPECIAL NEEDS

For all CME inquiries or special needs, please contact elsevierCME@elsevier.com.

MEDICAL CLINICS OF NORTH AMERICA

FORTHCOMING ISSUES

May 2024
Patient Management with Stable Ischemic Heart Disease
Alexander Fanaroff and John W. Hirshfeld Jr, *Editors*

July 2024
Allergy and Immunology
Andrew Lutzkanin and Kristen M. Lutzkanin, *Editors*

September 2024
Newer Outpatient Therapies and Treatments
Douglas Paauw, *Editor*

RECENT ISSUES

January 2024
Adolescent Undiagnosed and Rare Diseases
Heather Toth, Robert M. Kliegman and Brett Bordini, *Editors*

November 2023
Current Challenges and New Directions in Preventive Medicine
Marie Krousel-Wood, *Editor*

September 2023
Vascular Medicine
Geno J. Merli and Raghu Kolluri, *Editors*

Contributors

CONSULTING EDITOR

JACK ENDE, MD, MACP
The Schaeffer Professor of Medicine, Perelman School of Medicine, University of Pennsylvania, Philadelphia, Pennsylvania

EDITOR

SUSAN TUDDENHAM, MD, MPH
Associate Professor, Department of Medicine, Division of Infectious Diseases, Johns Hopkins University, Baltimore, Maryland

AUTHORS

KEVIN L. ARD, MD, MPH
Assistant Professor of Medicine, Harvard Medical School, Division of Infectious Diseases, Massachusetts General Hospital, Boston, Massachusetts

LINDLEY A. BARBEE, MD, MPH
Clinical Team Lead, Division of STD Prevention, Centers for Disease Control and Prevention, Atlanta, Georgia

LUIS F. BARROSO II, MD
Associate Professor, Department of Medicine, Section on Infectious Diseases, Wake Forest University School of Medicine, Winston-Salem, North Carolina

TERESA A. BATTEIGER, MD, MS
Assistant Professor of Medicine, Indiana University School of Medicine, Indianapolis, Indiana

KEOSHA T. BOND, EdD, MPH, CHES
Assistant Medical Professor, Department of Community Health and Social Medicine, CUNY School of Medicine, New York, New York; Faculty Fellow, Center for Interdisciplinary Research on AIDS at Yale University, Yale University School of Public Health, New Haven, Connecticut

CHASE A. CANNON, MD, MPH
Assistant Professor, Department of Medicine, Division of Allergy and Infectious Diseases, University of Washington, Public Health–Seattle and King County, Seattle, Washington

JOSEPH CHERABIE, MD, MSc
Assistant Professor, Department of Medicine, Division of Infectious Diseases, Washington University in St. Louis School of Medicine, St. Louis, Missouri

A.C. DEMIDONT, MD
Principal Medical Scientist, Gilead Sciences, Inc, HIV Treatment Medical Affairs, Foster City, California

ELIZABETH A. GILLIAMS, MD, MSc
Assistant Professor, Division of Infectious Diseases, Johns Hopkins School of Medicine, Johns Hopkins Bayview Medical Center, Baltimore, Maryland

SHAUNA GUNARATNE, MD, MPH
Diploma in Tropical Medicine and Hygiene; Assistant Professor, Division of Infectious Diseases, Columbia University Irving Medical Center, New York, New York

MATTHEW M. HAMILL, MBChB, PhD
Assistant Professor, Division of Infectious Diseases, Johns Hopkins School of Medicine, Johns Hopkins Bayview Medical Center, Baltimore, Maryland

DONALD HONG, MD
Assistant Professor, Department of Medicine, Division of Infectious Diseases, Washington University in St. Louis School of Medicine, St. Louis, Missouri

ZACHARY LORENZ, MD
Resident, Department of Medicine, Johns Hopkins School of Medicine, Johns Hopkins Bayview Medical Center, Baltimore, Maryland

ANDREW MACDONALD-LY, PharmD, AAHIVP
Consultant Pharmacist, Gilead Sciences, Inc, HIV Global Medical Affairs, Foster City, California

KENNETH H. MAYER, MD
Division of Infectious Diseases, The Fenway Institute, Fenway Health, Professor, Harvard Medical School, Beth Israel Deaconess Medical Center, Boston, Massachusetts

STEPHANIE E. MCLAUGHLIN, MD, MPH
Infectious Disease Physician, Acting Instructor, University of Washington, Seattle, Washington

CANDICE J. MCNEIL, MD, MPH
Associate Professor, Department of Medicine, Section on Infectious Diseases, Wake Forest University School of Medicine, Winston-Salem, North Carolina

JACOB MCLEAN, DO
Post-doctoral Research Fellow, Division of Infectious Diseases, Columbia University Irving Medical Center, New York, New York

CAROLINE MITCHELL, MD, MPH
Associate Professor, Department of Obstetrics and Gynecology, Harvard Medical School, Boston, Massachusetts

MASAYO NISHIYAMA, RN, DNP
Nurse Manager, Denver Sexual Health Clinic, Public Health Institute at Denver Health, Denver, Colorado

OLUYOMI A. OBAFEMI, MD, MPH
Medical Director, Denver Sexual Health Clinic, Public Health Institute at Denver Health, Denver, Colorado; Assistant Professor, Department of Family Medicine, University of Colorado Denver, Aurora, Colorado

LAURA A.S. QUILTER, MD, MPH
Medical Officer, Division of STD Prevention, Centers for Disease Control and Prevention, Atlanta, Georgia

ASA E. RADIX, MD, PhD, MPH
Associate Professor, Department of Epidemiology, Columbia University Mailman School of Public Health, New York, New York; Faculty Fellow, Center for Interdisciplinary Research on AIDS at Yale University, Yale School of Public Health, New Haven, Connecticut

MEENA S. RAMCHANDANI, MD, MPH
Associate Professor, Department of Medicine, Division of Allergy and Infectious Diseases, University of Washington, Public Health–Seattle and King County, Seattle, Washington

HILARY E. RENO, MD, PhD
Professor, Department of Medicine, Division of Infectious Diseases, Washington University in St. Louis School of Medicine, St. Louis, Missouri

CORNELIS A. RIETMEIJER, MD, PhD
Rietmeijer Consulting, Denver, Colorado

SARAH E. ROWAN, MD
Associate Director of HIV/STI Prevention and Control, Public Health Institute at Denver Health, Denver, Colorado; Associate Professor, Division of Infectious Diseases, Department of Medicine, University of Colorado Denver, Aurora, Colorado

JACK D. SOBEL, MD
Professor, Department of Medicine, Division of Infectious Diseases, Wayne State University, Detroit, Michigan

SANCTA B. ST. CYR, MD, MPH
Medical Officer, Division of STD Prevention, Centers for Disease Control and Prevention, Atlanta, Georgia

SUSAN TUDDENHAM, MD, MPH
Associate Professor, Department of Medicine, Division of Infectious Diseases, Johns Hopkins University, Baltimore, Maryland

KAREN A. WENDEL, MD
Director of HIV/STI Prevention and Control, Public Health Institute at Denver Health, Denver, Colorado; Assistant Professor of Medicine, Division of Infectious Diseases, Department of Medicine, University of Colorado Denver, Aurora, Colorado

KIMBERLY WORKOWSKI, MD
Professor, Department of Medicine, Division of Infectious Diseases, Emory University School of Medicine, Atlanta, Georgia

GOLSA M. YAZDY, MD
Assistant Professor, Department of Gynecology and Obstetrics, Johns Hopkins University, Baltimore, Maryland

JASON ZUCKER, MD, MS
Assistant Professor, Division of Infectious Diseases, Columbia University Irving Medical Center, New York, New York

Contents

Foreword: Sexually Transmitted Infections: Medicine in Its Fullest xv

Jack Ende

Preface: Sexually Transmitted Infections xvii

Susan Tuddenham

Sexual Health and Well-Being: A Framework to Guide Care 241

Keosha T. Bond and Asa E. Radix

Although the acceptance of sex positivity centering pleasure and justice has grown, clinical and public health strategies for sexually transmitted infection management have remained focused on risk and adverse outcomes. To promote sex-positive health care practice in clinical settings and beyond, health care practitioners should use an integrated, patient-centered approach to sexual health. These strategies include initiating discussions, continued sexual health education, providing informative material for patients, and knowledge of different communication strategies. Patient–provider interactions might be enhanced by using such methods.

Taking a Sexual History: Best Practices 257

Donald Hong, Joseph Cherabie, and Hilary E. Reno

Recognizing the holistic definitions of sexual health, health-care providers must approach sexual health history taking with sensitivity, inclusivity, and a trauma-informed perspective. Many versions of what a sexual history should look like exist but certain principles are commonly found. Education of health-care providers on sexual history taking can involve reviewing the components of the sexual history but should also include the importance of using nonstigmatizing language, having a patient-centered approach, and practicing trauma-informed and culturally sensitive care.

A Practical Approach to Sexually Transmitted Infection Screening for the Primary Care Clinician 267

Kevin L. Ard and Kenneth H. Mayer

Sexually transmitted infections (STIs) are commonly encountered in primary care. The Centers for Disease Control and Prevention and the US Preventive Services Task Force have both issued guidelines about screening for chlamydia, gonorrhea, syphilis, and HIV. By eliciting a sexual history, understanding their patients' anatomy, and considering factors which may increase the likelihood of STIs and their sequelae, clinicians can implement a practical, evidence-based approach to STI screening.

The Management of Gonorrhea in the Era of Emerging Antimicrobial Resistance: What Primary Care Clinicians Should Know **279**

Laura A.S. Quilter, Sancta B. St. Cyr, and Lindley A. Barbee

Gonorrhea rates continue to rise in the United States and *Neisseria gonorrhoeae's* propensity to develop resistance to all therapies used for treatment has complicated the management of gonorrhea. Ceftriaxone is the only remaining highly effective recommended regimen for gonococcal treatment and few new anti-gonococcal antimicrobials are being developed. The 2021 CDC STI Treatment Guidelines increased the dose of ceftriaxone to 500 mg (1 g if $\geq$ 150 kg) for uncomplicated infections. It is recommended that all clinicians should be aware of antimicrobial resistant gonorrhea and be able to appropriately manage any suspected gonorrhea treatment failure case.

Mycoplasma genitalium: Key Information for the Primary Care Clinician **297**

Oluyomi A. Obafemi, Sarah E. Rowan, Masayo Nishiyama, and Karen A. Wendel

Mycoplasma genitalium (MG) is an emerging sexually transmitted infection, which appears to be a cause of urethritis and cervicitis and has been associated with pelvic inflammatory disease (PID), epididymitis, proctitis, infertility, complications during pregnancy, and human immunodeficiency virus (HIV) transmission. Three Food and Drug Administration (FDA) approved tests are available. Testing should be focused to avoid inappropriate antibiotic use. The Centers of Disease Control and Prevention (CDC) guidelines recommend testing for persistent male urethritis, cervicitis, and proctitis and state that testing should be considered in cases of PID. Testing is also recommended for sexual contacts of patients with MG. Testing is not recommended in asymptomatic patients, including pregnant patients, who do not have a history of MG exposure. Although resistance-guided therapy is recommended, there are currently no FDA approved tests for MG macrolide resistance, and tests are not widely available in the United States. The CDC recommends 2-step treatment with doxycycline followed by azithromycin or moxifloxacin. Moxifloxacin is recommended if resistance testing is unavailable or testing demonstrates macrolide resistance.

Herpes Simplex Virus: A Practical Guide to Diagnosis, Management, and Patient Counseling for the Primary Care Clinician **311**

Teresa A. Batteiger and Cornelis A. Rietmeijer

Genital herpes is a chronic, lifelong sexually transmitted viral infection, which can cause recurrent, self-limited genital ulcers. It is caused by herpes simplex virus (HSV) type 1 and type 2 viruses. Genital HSV infection is a very prevalent STI, which causes self-limited, recurrent genital ulcers. Treatment decreases duration of symptoms and signs and can be provided as episodic or suppressive therapy. Genital herpes can have a substantial impact during pregnancy and on sexual health in general. Counseling on natural history, transmission, treatment, and management of sexual partners is an integral part of management of genital herpes.

Syphilis Serologies: A Practical Approach for the Primary Care Clinician **325**

Elizabeth A. Gilliams, Zachary Lorenz, and Matthew M. Hamill

Syphilis serology interpretation can be challenging even for experienced providers. This article reviews the staging of syphilis and the principles of syphilis serology testing, the algorithms used in diagnosis, and guidance for their use in monitoring the response to treatment. The authors illustrate these principles through a series of clinical scenarios and describe the rationale behind the management approaches.

Proctitis: An Approach to the Symptomatic Patient 339

Candice J. McNeil, Luis F. Barroso II, and Kimberly Workowski

Proctitis is an inflammatory condition of the distal rectum that can be associated with common sexually transmitted infections (STIs), such as gonorrhea, chlamydia, and syphilis. For persons presenting with ulcerative findings on examination, in addition to syphilis, Mpox, lymphogranuloma venereum, and herpes simplex virus should be in the differential. Providers should also be aware that there are evolving data to support a role for *Mycoplasma genitalium* in proctitis. Performing a comprehensive history, clinical evaluation including anoscopy, and rectal nucleic amplification STI testing may be useful in identifying the cause of proctitis and targeting treatment.

Update on Mpox: What the Primary Care Clinician Should Know 355

Jacob McLean, Shauna Gunaratne, and Jason Zucker

Mpox is a viral infection, which primarily caused sporadic outbreaks in West and Central Africa until causing a global epidemic in 2022. The disease has disproportionately affected people with human immunodeficiency virus and men who have sex with men. Transmission is through close physical contact, including sexual contact. Infection presents with a characteristic rash, with frequent anogenital involvement—polymerase chain reaction of skin lesions is diagnostic. Vaccination is available for primary prevention and postexposure prophylaxis. Treatment consists of supportive care, with antiviral medications available via clinical trials and/or for patients with severe disease.

Recurrent Infectious Vaginitis: A Practical Approach for the Primary Care Clinician 373

Golsa M. Yazdy, Caroline Mitchell, Jack D. Sobel, and Susan Tuddenham

Recurrent infectious vaginitis can lead to significant morbidity, patient frustration, and health care costs. The most common causes are bacterial vaginosis (BV) and vulvovaginal candidiasis (VVC); however, other infectious and noninfectious etiologies should be considered in patients with recurrent symptoms. A detailed history and physical examination with appropriate testing at the time of symptoms is critical to establishing a correct diagnosis. Management options for recurrent BV and VVC are limited. Complex cases including those with atypical symptoms, negative testing for common causes, refractory symptoms despite appropriate therapy or recurrences during suppressive therapy will require referral to specialist care.

Sexual Health Care for Transgender and Gender Diverse People 393

Kevin L. Ard, Andrew MacDonald-Ly, and A.C Demidont

The proportion of people who identify as transgender and gender diverse (TGD) is increasing. Health care for TGD people, including sexual health care, must affirm and respect patients' gender identities and expressions.

Here, the authors outline strategies to make health care settings more welcoming to and inclusive of TGD people and describe concrete steps to improve sexual health care for TGD populations.

On The Horizon: Novel Approaches to Sexually Transmitted Infection Prevention **403**

Chase A. Cannon, Stephanie E. McLaughlin, and Meena S. Ramchandani

Rates of sexually transmitted infections (STIs), especially cases of infectious and congenital syphilis, are increasing in the United States. Novel strategies for STI prevention are being explored and include doxycycline post-exposure prophylaxis and the potential utility of vaccines against gonorrhea. Self-collection of samples and point of care testing for STI are increasingly being employed in a variety of settings. Both can improve uptake of screening and lead to earlier detection and treatment of incident STI in target populations. Overcoming existing regulatory issues and optimizing implementation of current evidence-based strategies will be key to maximizing future STI prevention efforts. Here we provide an update for primary care providers on selected new strategies for STI prevention either currently available or under development for possible future use.

Foreword
Sexually Transmitted Infections: Medicine in Its Fullest

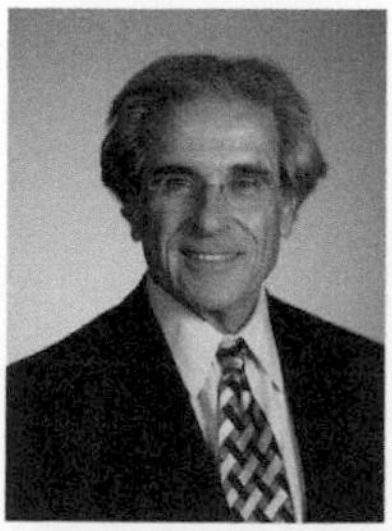

Jack Ende, MD, MACP
Consulting Editor

As far back as ancient times, sexually transmitted infections (STIs) have been part of the human condition. Records from ancient Egypt, Greece, and Rome depict outbreaks of gonorrhea and syphilis. The Middle Ages saw epidemics of both these diseases, which, of course, were untreatable then, leading to stigmatization, isolation, and shame, accompaniments of STIs that persist to this day. As populations became more mobile, initially with ocean voyages in the time of Christopher Columbus, and all the way up to modern times with air travel, STIs spread in both senses of the word: from patient to patient and from continent to continent. Now, of course, several STIs (though not all) are treatable, while asymptomatic latency periods and disregard for safe sexual practices challenge our best efforts at control. This is especially the case in underserved or stigmatized populations, and in parts of the world that are considered resource poor.

What is the lesson we can learn from medicine's eternal struggle to prevent and treat, if not eliminate, STIs? I believe, and I trust our guest editor and authors would agree, we need to view STIs as part of the human condition. For as long as humans have engaged and will continue to engage in sexual activity, we will be faced with STIs. Is this a fatalistic or nihilistic lesson? Hardly. As so clearly laid out in this issue of *Medical Clinics of North America*, there is so much that can be done, from more effective treatments, to evidence-based strategies for screening and prevention, and to more enlightened paradigms for patient-centered, inclusive approaches to care for patients with STIs.

STIs represent medicine in its full historical, geopolitical, socioeconomic, and population-based context. If ever there was a field demanding of our attention, this is one.

Med Clin N Am 108 (2024) xv–xvi
https://doi.org/10.1016/j.mcna.2023.10.005

Credit goes to Dr Susan Tuddenham for bringing together the expert authors and identifying the topics that make this issue of *Medical Clinics of North America* so important for practicing physicians and other health care providers.

Jack Ende, MD, MACP
Perelman School of Medicine
of the University of Pennsylvania
Philadelphia, PA, USA

E-mail address:
jack.ende@pennmedicine.upenn.edu

Preface
Sexually Transmitted Infections

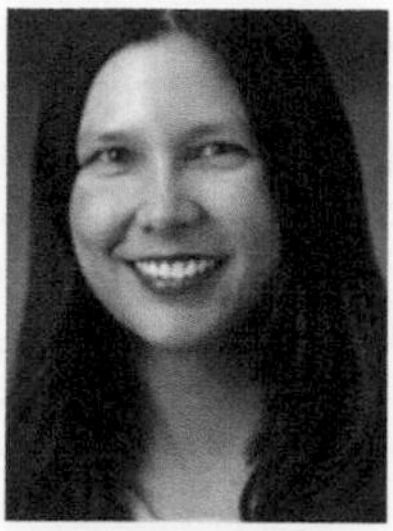

Susan Tuddenham, MD, MPH
Editor

Sexually Transmitted Infections (STIs) are associated with significant stigma and can lead to debilitating symptoms and poor obstetric and reproductive outcomes. Asymptomatic infections can fuel transmission, and left untreated, may lead to significant sequelae for the individual patient.[1] Unfortunately, STIs are on the rise in the United States, and concerns for developing drug resistance and new emerging pathogens may complicate management.[2] Over time, and with decreased availability of dedicated STI clinics, patients have increasingly sought care for STIs in primary care settings.[3] Moreover, these settings offer important opportunities to engage patients to improve their sexual health and provide STI screening to eligible asymptomatic individuals. Thus, primary care providers (PCPs) are on the front lines of the fight against STIs.[3] This issue of *Medical Clinics of North America* aims to educate PCPs on some of the most important issues in STI management. Our goals are not to comprehensively review and address all aspects of every possible STI, nor to recapitulate the excellent national guidelines[1] that already exist. Rather, we have chosen specific topics to highlight key new information or explore common STI management dilemmas encountered by PCPs, striving to provide practical guidance directly relevant to their practice.

STI rates have continued to rise in the face of traditional approaches to prevention and care, which often focus exclusively on negative health outcomes and fear of danger or disease. In the article in the issue, "Sexual Health and Well-Being: A Framework to Guide Care," Bond and Radix introduce PCPs to an alternative, more positive framework with which to approach patients, which is rooted in the concept of sexual health. Despite the importance of such approaches, providers often lack education on how practically to apply these concepts to their own practice. Therefore, the article in the series, "Taking a Sexual History: Best Practices" by Hong and colleagues, provides information on how, informed by holistic definitions of sexual health and other key concepts, providers can best implement an approach to sexual history taking that

Med Clin N Am 108 (2024) xvii–xix
https://doi.org/10.1016/j.mcna.2023.10.004 medical.theclinics.com
0025-7125/24/© 2023 Published by Elsevier Inc.

is sensitive and inclusive. The article, "Sexual Health Care for Transgender and Gender Diverse People" by Ard, MacDonald-Ly and Demidont, provides additional details on sexual health in transgender and gender-diverse populations, who may be disproportionately impacted by STIs.

Other articles in the series provide guidance on STI screening (which is critical to interrupting transmission and decreasing STI rates as well as the sequelae of untreated infection in asymptomatic patients), discuss approaches to symptomatic proctitis, detail key aspects of care for genital Herpes Simplex Virus, cover interpretation of syphilis serologies (a perennial source of confusion for general practitioners and specialists alike), and review clinical syndromes, diagnosis, and current recommendations for management of *Mycoplasma genitalium*, an emerging STI of considerable interest for which a lack of robust data and drug resistance create distinct challenges. Mpox rates have declined, but new outbreaks have highlighted the importance of awareness of this new infection for PCPs; the article on mpox details currently available information, including guidance on first steps to take in evaluation and management of suspected cases. Our article on recurrent infectious vaginitis explains how practically to approach diagnosis and initial management of this condition (for which STIs are on the differential). In addition, antimicrobial resistance in gonorrhea threatens the future of STI control. In January 2023, concerning reports of multidrug-resistant gonorrhea in the United States emerged.[4] Given that, if current trends continue, PCPs may well be among the first to encounter gonococcal drug resistance or even treatment failure to first-line recommended antibiotics, the article focused on gonorrhea provides education geared toward a primary care audience, including specific guidance on what to do in cases of suspected gonococcal treatment failure.

Last, as rising case rates show, new and innovative approaches to STI prevention are desperately needed. Some of these, such as doxycycline-PEP, are already being implemented in select areas in the United States. Others may be further away but hold promise. The article in the series, "On the Horizon: Novel Approaches to STI Prevention," by Cannon and colleagues highlights some of these emerging biomedical and testing approaches. From the clinical standpoint, reducing incidence and managing STIs require informed, patient-centered, and inclusive approaches to sexual health care. We hope that these articles provide practical, useful guidance to aid PCPs as they provide these needed services.

CONFLICT OF INTEREST/DISCLOSURES

Susan Tuddenham has been a consultant for BioFire Diagnostics, Roche Molecular Diagnostics, and Luca Biologics, receives royalties from UpToDate, and has received speaker honoraria from Roche Molecular Diagnostics and Medscape/WebMD. She participates in research supported by donation of test kits to her academic institution by Hologic.

FUNDING

Susan Tuddenham is supported by grants from the Gates foundation and the National Institutes of Health (R01DK13085, R21AI156765, R21AI168984, U54EB007958).

Susan Tuddenham, MD, MPH
Department of Medicine
Division of Infectious Diseases
Johns Hopkins University
5200 Eastern Avenue
MFL Center Tower, Suite 381
Baltimore, MD 21224, USA

E-mail address:
Studden1@jhmi.edu

REFERENCES

1. Workowski KA, Bachmann LH, Chan PA, et al. Sexually transmitted infections treatment guidelines, 2021. MMWR Recomm Rep 2021;70(4):1–187.
2. Centers for Disease Control Sexually Transmitted Disease Surveillance 2021. Available at: https://www.cdc.gov/std/statistics/2021/default.htm. Accessed October 4, 2023.
3. Barrow RY, Ahmed F, Bolan GA, et al. Recommendations for providing quality sexually transmitted diseases clinical services, 2020. MMWR Recomm Rep 2020;68(5):1–20.
4. Press Release Massachusetts Department of Public Health. "Department of Public Health announces first cases of concerning gonorrhea strain." Available at: https://www.mass.gov/news/department-of-public-health-announces-first-cases-of-concerning-gonorrhea-strain#:~:text=Boston%20%E2%80%94%20The%20Department%20of%20Public,indicate%20a%20similar%20drug%20response. Accessed October 4, 2023.

Sexual Health and Well-Being: A Framework to Guide Care

Keosha T. Bond, EdD, MPH, CHES[a,b,*], Asa E. Radix, MD, PhD, MPH[b,c]

KEYWORDS

- Sex-positive health care • Pleasure • Sexuality • Sexuality education
- Sexual health promotion • Sexual rights • Patient–provider communication
- Structural competency

KEY POINTS

- Sexual health should not only be discussed in relation to sexually transmitted infections (STIs/HIV) and unintended pregnancy but also to promote pleasure and address structural challenges to health care engagement.
- Sexual health is an important area of primary care that is often neglected in clinical settings and medical training. Many health care professionals lack training and knowledge to provide sex-positive health care.
- A sex-positive approach to sexual health care and well-being includes the prioritization of pleasure and integration of structural competence practices in clinical settings.

WHAT IS SEXUAL HEALTH?

Sex positivity and more broadly sexual well-being have become increasingly important on the global health agenda in recent years, although the focus on negative outcomes still dominates discussions of sexuality, provision of sexual health care, and management of sexually transmitted infections (STIs).[1] This shift in the narrative around sexual health calls for a pleasure-based approach, which is fundamental to reducing stigma related to sexuality and addressing elements such as consent, privacy, and communication that contribute to sexual health and well-being. Sexual health, as defined by the World Health Organization, is

> *...a state of physical, emotional, mental, and social well-being in relation to sexuality; it is not merely the absence of disease, dysfunction, or infirmity. Sexual*

[a] Department of Community Health and Social Medicine, CUNY School of Medicine, 160 Convent Avenue, Harris Hall, New York, NY 10031, USA; [b] Center for Interdisciplinary Research on AIDS at Yale University, Yale University School of Public Health, 135 College Street, Suite 200, New Haven, CT 06510-2483, USA; [c] Department of Epidemiology, Columbia University Mailman School of Public Health, 722 West 168th Street, New York, NY 10032, USA
* Coressponding author. Department of Community Health and Social Medicine, CUNY School of Medicine, 160 Convent Avenue, Harris Hall, New York, NY 10031.
E-mail address: kbond@med.cuny.edu

Med Clin N Am 108 (2024) 241–255
https://doi.org/10.1016/j.mcna.2023.10.001
0025-7125/24/
medical.theclinics.com

health requires a positive and respectful approach to sexuality and sexual relationships, as well as the possibility of having pleasurable and safe sexual experiences, free of coercion, discrimination, and violence. For sexual health to be attained and maintained, the sexual rights of all persons must be respected, protected, and fulfilled.[2]

This concept of sexual health can help health care providers (HCPs) (as well as researchers, educators, and policymakers) recognize positive sexuality and sexual experiences as important health outcomes.

PLEASURE-INCLUSIVE VERSUS EXCLUSIVELY RISK-BASED APPROACHES TO SEXUAL HEALTH AND BEHAVIORS

Sexual health and well-being extend beyond the simple absence of adverse outcomes such as STIs and include a culture where each person is guided in having a safe and pleasurable sexual life. As sexual health is an important component of a person's overall health, discussions about sexuality beyond the act of sex cannot be overlooked or discounted. Without a thorough assessment of sexuality, which underlies significant behaviors, experiences, and has implications outside of sexual acts, sexual health cannot be well-defined, understood, or operationalized. For sexual well-being to be attained and maintained, it is critical for the sexual rights of all persons to be respected, protected, and fulfilled in clinical settings.

However, too often, clinical (as well as public health) approaches to sexual health care and prevention and management of STIs focus exclusively on negative health outcomes and the labeling of sexual behaviors as risk factors while ignoring other aspects of sexuality.[1,3] Within an exclusively risk-based approach, discussions of sexual pleasure are always absent, and patient–provider conversations instead focus solely on risks, pathogens, and testing (see **Table 1**).[4]

Yet, there is no evidence that a sex-negative or risk-based approach to health care and safer sex promotion leads to safer sexual behaviors.

In reality, people engage in sexual activity for a variety of reasons, including bonding with others, love and affection, cultural expectations, economic necessity, easing stress, social contracts such as marriage and procreation, and importantly, sexual pleasure. Sexual pleasure is one of the main factors driving sexual behaviors. The World Association of Sexual Health (WAS) recently adopted sexual pleasure as an essential component of sexual health, defining it as "the physical and/or psychological satisfaction and enjoyment derived from shared or solitary erotic experiences, including thoughts, fantasies, dreams, emotions, and feelings."[5] In their statements on sexual rights, WAS stressed the importance of pleasurable, satisfying, and safe sexual experiences (**Box 1**).[6] A growing body of research shows that sexual pleasure is essential to overall health, mental health, sexual health, well-being, and rights and that it can even lead to health improvements.[5]

The strategy of combining pleasure, sexual health promotion, and STI/HIV prevention is gaining momentum as it has been shown to generate and sustain interest in sexual health promotion among vulnerable populations while encouraging safe sexual health practices. A recent meta-analysis of 33 unique interventions targeting STIs and safer sex practices from 2005 to 2020 found that prioritizing pleasure, rather than the fear of danger or disease, increases the likelihood of safer sex practices.[7] Sexual health programs that include sexual desire and sexual pleasure were found to improve knowledge and attitudes around sex and increase condom use, as compared with those that did not.[7] Although more research is needed to determine the best ways to incorporate sexual pleasure to achieve sexual health for various outcomes

Table 1
Risk-based approach versus pleasure-based approach in sexual health

Pleasure-Based Approach	Risk-Based Approach
Messages are centered on sexuality as a source of pleasure and well-being for all individuals, and the importance of attaining ideal sexual experiences is emphasized.	Solely emphasizes risks of HIV, STIs, unintended pregnancy, and other undesirable consequences of sexual activity in all messages.
Recognizes that sexual pleasure is the primary reason why people engage in sexual activity and that pleasure determines how we make sexual decisions.	Does not recognize the significance of understanding why people engage in sexual activity, including to experience pleasure or to appreciate each other's company.
Actively promotes pleasure as a crucial ingredient for individuals to engage in safer sexual practice and use HIV/STI prevention methods (ie, regular screening, PrEP, PEP, condoms).	Reinforces fear-based messaging or shame as the primary motive for people to use sexual protection, for example, if you have sex without a condom, you will catch HIV, so wear a condom.
Encourages reflection and conversation about the connections between sexual pleasure, sexual health, and sexual rights such as self-determination, consent, privacy, safety, communication, diversity, negotiation, and confidence.	Exclusively addresses the medical and biological aspects pertaining to the unintended consequences, encompassing symptoms, diagnostic procedures, and therapeutic interventions.
Advocates for the dissemination of messages that normalize discussions surrounding sexual pleasure within the context of sexual health and sexual rights. Encourages development of trusted patient–provider relationships that encourage bidirectional communication, including accurate information regarding STIs, prevention, and treatment.	Maintain traditional views of sexuality that can be a source of fuel for the stigma that surrounds sexuality during the process of offering education, counseling, and information to patients or evaluating the condition of a patient.

and populations, a pleasure-inclusive sexual health approach holds promise for increasing patients' sexual self-esteem, sexual self-confidence, and safe choices (**Table 1**). Importantly, a pleasure-based approach does not mean STI adverse effects, prevention and treatment are not accurately communicated; rather it supports the development of trusted patient–provider relationships that encourages bidirectional communication of this information.

BARRIERS TO SEXUAL HEALTH SERVICES

Stigma and Shame

Seeking and engaging in sexual health services is important to overall health and well-being. However, multiple barriers exist that can prevent individuals accessing these services, the most predominant of which has been stigma and shame. Sexual pleasure has been viewed as a threat to social, political, and religious order throughout history. Discourse around sex in medical, academic, and clinical settings focused solely on disease, risk, and shame can contribute to stigma not only related to STI/HIV acquisition but all aspects of sexual health and well-being.[8] Factors such as trepidation about social capital, negative perceptions surrounding STI/HIV, and concerns about personal reputation may make patients less likely to engage with needed sexual health

Box 1
World Association for Sexual Health's Declaration on Sexual Pleasure

In recognition that sexual pleasure is a fundamental part of sexual health and sexual rights, the World Association for Sexual Health:

RECOGNIZES that:

Sexual pleasure is the physical and/or psychological satisfaction and enjoyment derived from shared or solitary erotic experiences, including thoughts, fantasies, dreams, emotions, and feelings. Self-determination, consent, safety, privacy, confidence, and the ability to communicate and negotiate sexual relations are key enabling factors for pleasure to contribute to sexual health and well-being. Sexual pleasure should be exercised within the context of sexual rights, particularly the rights to equality and nondiscrimination, autonomy and bodily integrity, the right to the highest attainable standard of health and freedom of expression. The experiences of human sexual pleasure are diverse and sexual rights ensure that pleasure is a positive experience for all concerned and not obtained by violating other people's human rights and well-being.

DECLARES that:

1. The possibility of having pleasurable and safe sexual experiences free of discrimination, coercion, and violence is a fundamental part of sexual health and well-being for all
2. Access to sources of sexual pleasure is part of human experience and subjective well-being;
3. Sexual pleasure is a fundamental part of sexual rights as a matter of human rights;
4. Sexual pleasure includes the possibility of diverse sexual experiences;
5. Sexual pleasure shall be integrated into education, health promotion and service delivery, research and advocacy in all parts of the world;
6. The programmatic inclusion of sexual pleasure to meet individuals' needs, aspirations, and realities ultimately contributes to global health and sustainable development and it should require comprehensive, immediate, and sustainable action.

URGES all governments, international intergovernmental and non-governmental organizations, academic institutions, health and education authorities, the media, private sector actors, and society at large, and particularly, all member organizations of the World Association for Sexual Health to:

A. Promote sexual pleasure in law and policy as a fundamental part of sexual health and well-being, grounded in the principles of sexual rights as human rights, including self-determination, nondiscrimination, privacy, bodily integrity, and equality;
B. Ensure that comprehensive sexuality education addresses sexual pleasure in an inclusive, evidence-informed, and rights-based manner tailored to people's diverse capacities and needs across the life span, in order to allow experiences of informed, self-determined, respectful, and safe sexual pleasure;
C. Guarantee that sexual pleasure is integral to sexual health care services provision, and that sexual health services are accessible, affordable, acceptable, and free from stigma, discrimination, and prosecution;
D. Enhance the development of rights-based, evidence-informed knowledge of the benefits of sexual pleasure as part of well-being, including rights-based funding resources, research methodologies, and dissemination of knowledge to address the role of sexual pleasure in individual and public health;
E. Reaffirm the global, national, community, interpersonal, and individual commitments to recognition of the diversity in sexual pleasure experiences respecting human rights of all people and supported by consistent, evidence-informed policy and practices, interpersonal behavior, and collective action.

From the Global Advisory Board for Sexual Health and Wellbeing (2016). Working definition of Sexual Pleasure. Retrieved from https://www.gab-shw.org/our-work/working-definition-of-sexual-pleasure.

services.[9] In a study with patients exploring physician-inspired shame and guilt, more than half of the respondents reported experiencing shame over their sexual habits. The study found 45% of patients who experienced shame reacted negatively by either terminating treatment with, avoiding, or lying to their physician as a result of the incident.[10] In addition to avoiding "stigma by association," marginalized communities frequently opt not to seek sexual health care services because they do not want to face stigma from care professionals about their sexual practices as they pertain to their gender and sexual identities.[11] For example, people who are most vulnerable may be hesitant to seek care because they do not want to be stigmatized as promiscuous because they seek sexual health services in health care clinics.

Cultural Mistrust

Cultural mistrust is another obstacle to sexual health service interest and utilization among vulnerable, marginalized communities.[12] Many people delay obtaining medical care because they lack trust in the health care system or are hesitant to build trustworthy connections with doctors; others opt to avoid dealing with the health care system entirely.[12] This mistrust stems from historical events, ongoing biases within the system, and the stigmatization of groups based on their race/ethnicity, gender, sexual orientation, and economic status, all of which make it difficult for marginalized communities who are disproportionately affected by adverse health outcomes to seek health care.[13,14] Providing health care that is more holistic, and embraces the entire person, as opposed to reductionist or focusing solely on specific body systems and components is essential to combating, stigma, discrimination, and oppressive cultural and societal norms associated with creating barriers to engagement in sexual health services and practices.[15–17]

Poor Access

Access to patient-centered services is essential; however, individuals may experience challenges accessing welcoming and knowledgeable providers, especially if they are members of minoritized and stigmatized groups, including transgender and gender diverse individuals,[18] sex workers,[19] and even the elderly.[20] Practical concerns, such as geographic distance and lack of transportation, can result in individuals not having adequate access to sexual health services.

Before interventions can be undertaken to reduce barriers to sexual health services, clinicians must be attuned to the patient's circumstances and past experiences with health care.

BEYOND SEXUALLY TRANSMITTED INFECTIONS: SEX AND THE BIDIRECTIONAL ASSOCIATIONS BETWEEN MENTAL AND PHYSICAL HEALTH

Complex and bidirectional associations exist between physical and mental health, and these relationships have important influences on sexual health and more specifically sexual functioning. Understanding these relationships is essential to optimizing quality of life and underscores the need to use a holistic approach that includes discussions of sexual health and pleasure in all aspects of health care.

In 2018, almost half of Americans aged more than 20 years were living with cardiovascular disease (CVD), with rates increasing by age.[21] Both existence of and underlying risk factors for CVD (eg, diabetes mellitus, dyslipidemia, and hypertension) as well as the medications use to treat them (eg, beta blockers, angiotensin-converting enzyme inhibitors and thiazide diuretics, among others) have known associations with sexual dysfunction.[22–26]

Similar interactions with mental and physical health and sexual function are seen for many other physical conditions, such as cancer, chronic kidney disease, chronic obstructive pulmonary disease, and HIV. Physical health conditions on their own can directly result in anxiety, depression, and other mood disorders.[23] Even more challenging is that the primary treatments for some mental health conditions, for example, selective serotonin reuptake inhibitors and antipsychotics can further exacerbate impediments in sexual function, desire, and satisfaction.[27] Often patients will not report these symptoms or side effects unless directly questioned so that the known prevalence of these associations is underreported.[27] Research has shown that sexual dysfunction is often associated with mood disorders, even when these are untreated.[28] These complex bidirectional relationships underscore the need for clinicians to conduct a comprehensive assessment of physical and mental health conditions as well as to document all prescribed and nonprescribed (ie, over the counter) medications to understand all potential factors that may contribute to sexual health and well-being.

EMPHASIS ON WELL-BEING

The medicalization of social problems has ethical implications for practitioners providing sexual health care.[29] Physicians are trained to ask, "What is this patient's primary problem?" Although treating the patient's current concern is critical, it is also important to broaden the therapeutic emphasis to include approaches that maximize and reconnect patients with their sense of completeness, embodiment, health, and structural integrity. The concept of sexual well-being can be defined as the maintenance of physical, mental, and emotional balance, and stability, encompassing more than the lack of disease. This perspective situates sexual well-being within the realms of sexual pleasure and sexual justice, recognizing their collective significance in addressing the underlying factors contributing to sexual inequities.[30]

Physicians have a responsibility to strike a balance between their pursuit of patient care and respect for patient's autonomy and the realities of institutional and structural discrimination that patients face. Because HCPs are trained to treat individuals with sexual health problems or negative health outcomes, they may contribute to the replication of problematic trends in health care by ignoring structural barriers to care.[29] Learning to address these hurdles and incorporate language and behaviors in clinical settings that facilitate sexual health interviewing will become easier with practice. Although HCPs cannot change the variety of sociocultural and interpersonal factors in their patients' lives, they can help them understand the influence these circumstances may have on their sexual health. Clinicians and staff should be trained in culturally sensitive terminology, gender-affirming care, structural humility, and assessment of personal internal biases to improve patient interactions to build a clinical environment that reassures patients that the practice is confidential, safe, affirming, and nonjudgmental.

WHEN SHOULD SEXUAL HEALTH DISCUSSIONS BE INITIATED?

Pleasure-based conversations about sexual health can be integrated into different types of primary care visits and should not be relegated only to specific visit types (eg, only when a person presents with symptoms of an STI). Opportunities can arise during any health maintenance visit or follow-up for chronic conditions. Adverse effects, including on sexual health, should be disclosed when new medications are prescribed, as often they may not be apparent to the patient (eg, individual who initiates finasteride for androgenetic hair loss may not realize that this drug may cause sexual dysfunction). Clinicians should also discuss potential changes in sexual function that might occur with certain health conditions. For example, diabetes mellitus may be associated with low libido, erectile dysfunction, ejaculatory dysfunction, and painful receptive vaginal sex as a result of microvascular disease, nerve damage, immune dysregulation, and infection that can often be managed through close monitoring and effective treatment.[31] Sexual health and well-being should be discussed after during pregnancy, the postpartum period, menopause, and after genital (including anal) surgeries. Many patients may have concerns about the safety of reengaging in sexual activities after being hospitalized, and starting these conversations early is important to provide appropriate information and allay patient fears. Focusing on pleasure to help patients with illness-related sexual changes may improve not only sexual health but overall health.

RECOMMENDATIONS FOR CENTERING SEX-POSITIVE PATIENT CARE

Applying a sex-positive approach that encompasses both elements of structural competency and pleasure in clinical interactions can assist with addressing barriers to sexual health care engagement. Sex positivity is defined by the International Planned Parenthood Federation as "an attitude that celebrates sexuality as a part of life that can enhance happiness, bringing energy and celebration."[32] Combining structural competency with pleasure-based approaches may improve clinician sensitivity to social determinants of health, foster generative self-reflection, and open doors to patient solidarity. Here, we apply structural competency elements[33] with a pleasure-based approach to provide a framework for sex-positive health care (**Fig. 1**) and recommend the following.

1. Patient-centered and tailored approaches should recognize the structural elements influencing clinical interactions.

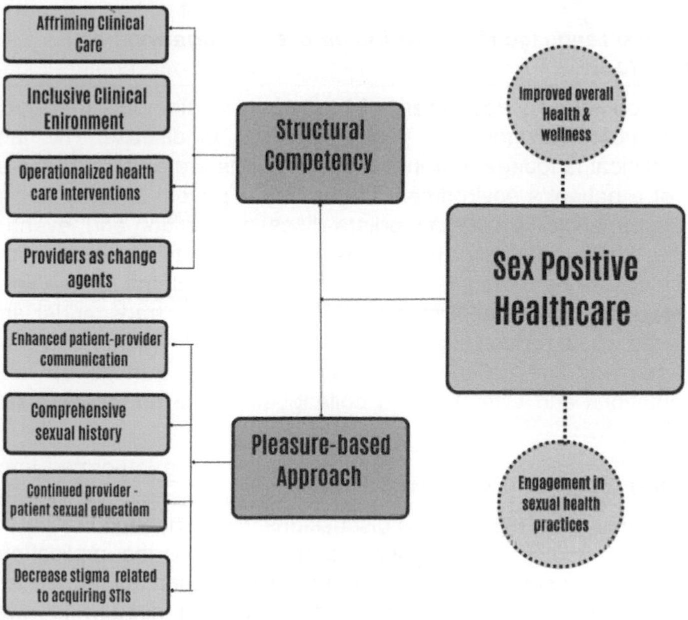

Fig. 1. Sex-positive health care framework.

2. Use extra-clinical language that is affirming over a judgmental and discriminatory tone.
3. Sexual wellness discussions begin with sexuality.
4. Incorporate models of sexual history taking that work best for your patients.

Patient-Centered and Tailored Approaches Should Recognize Structural Elements

Although the patient–provider relationship remains important, developments in the health care system show that a greater range of clinical, structural, and interpersonal factors can all influence the patient's experience. On a structural level, health care structures should provide calm welcoming spaces that accommodate patients' needs and offer inclusive resources and services. It is essential that patients can navigation through the system from intake to discharge. This means that when a patient enters your clinical setting, services begin. For example, the name and pronoun(s) that a transgender patient uses can be included in their electronic records to improve their experience in the clinical setting and minimized the risk of being misgendered and creating another barrier to sexual wellness discussions (see also Ard and colleagues[34] article on care for transgender and gender diverse populations and Cherabie and colleagues[35] article on sexual history taking in this issue). These structural elements support patient–provider relationships that promote communication on sexuality and intimacy to encourage patients to ask questions about sexual health (ie, inquiring about doxycycline post-exposure prophylaxis [Doxy-PEP] for STI prevention). Sex-positive messages with same- and different-gender couples, as well as persons of different ethnicities, gender expressions, and physical abilities, should be featured on posters, pamphlets, and other materials. Providers have a responsibility to establish a conducive environment that fosters a sense of ease for clients to openly discuss matters related to sexuality, free from any apprehension of being judged. This facilitates individuals in confidently exchanging and evaluating their sexual and reproductive health needs.

Use Extra-Clinical Language that Is Affirming over a Judgmental and Discriminatory Tone

Clinicians can construct a vocabulary of the structural elements that goes beyond the clinical symptoms, signs, and pathophysiology of disease. This language is called extra-clinical language. For instance, clinicians are able to observe how the "structure" of a patient's environment might limit a patient's ability to make decisions that are beneficial to their immediate disease condition and, eventually, their overall health. Using culturally appropriate terminology to convey pleasure could help sexual pleasure be more integrated within certain cultural and social contexts. For example, using gender neutral terms for anatomy for transgender and gender diverse patients would reduce stigma and support sexuality, autonomy, and individuality (also see Ard and colleagues article on care for transgender and gender diverse populations and Cherabie and colleagues article on sexual history taking in this issue).

Sexual Wellness Discussions Begin with Sexuality

To engage patients in sexual wellness discussions, HCPs need to cultivate structural humility by understanding their limitations and understand the implications of their explicit and implicit biases. This approach to communication acknowledges how unjust social determinants influence access to resources needed to make health changes and choices, such as the differential treatment patients receive from health care institutions and professionals based on race, gender, sexual orientation, class, or immigration status. In order to effectively help individuals in achieving sexual empowerment and experiencing sexual satisfaction, it is imperative for providers to possess a comprehensive understanding of sexuality, including sexual pleasure, as well as a familiarity with the prevalent physical and mental challenges encountered by clients across various sexual orientations and age groups. Health practitioners should pursue professional development opportunities to improve their skills in caring for transgender and gender nonconforming people. Although gender-affirming treatment is not always related to sexual health, sexual health providers should receive additional training in queer and trans health and provide these vital services (**Table 2** for educational resources).

Incorporate Models of Sexual History-Taking that Work Best for Patients

It is vital to incorporate regular inquiries regarding sexual well-being and pleasure. The determination of the impact of sex on patients' quality of life remains unknown in the absence of soliciting their perspectives. Without inquiring, it is impossible to ascertain the exact kind of sexual activities that contribute to an individual's pleasure nor can providers make assumptions on their prioritization of sexual functioning within the framework of their medical treatment.

The acquisition of a sexual history provides an opportunity to evaluate the various connections between sexual pleasure, sexual health, and sexual rights. There are three essential aspects during the assessment of sexual wellness with patients. What are your sexual wellness goals? What does the word "sex" mean to you? What types of sexual activities are significant for enhancing personal and mutual satisfaction within intimate relationships?

Table 2
Online sex-positive educational resources for health care providers

Area of Interest	Source	Link
Pleasure	The Pleasure Project	https://thepleasureproject.org
	American Sexual Health Association	https://www.ashasexualhealth.org
	Global Advisory Board for Sexual Health and Wellbeing	https://www.gab-shw.org
	National Coalition for Sexual Health	https://nationalcoalitionforsexualhealth.org/tools/for-healthcare-providers/compendium-of-sexual-reproductive-health-resources-for-healthcare-providers
	The Center for Sexual Pleasure and Health	https://thecsph.org
	The Pleasure Principal	https://thepleasureprincipal.org/resources/
Transgender Health	World Professional Association for Transgender Health	https://www.wpath.org
	Human Right Campaign Safer Sex for Trans-Bodies	https://www.hrc.org/resources/safer-sex-for-trans-bodies
	USCF Center for Transgender Health	https://prevention.ucsf.edu/transhealth/resources
Youth	Sex Positive Families	https://sexpositivefamilies.com
	National Sex Ed Conference	http://sexedconference.com/about-cse/

Table 3
Examples of sex-positive framing of questions for initiating sexual assessment

	Areas of Sexual Health History	Recommendations	Example Questions
Pleasure-based 5Ps	Partners	Ask questions about the patient's partner(s) without assumptions about the patient's sexual orientation, the gender identity of the patient or partners, or their relationship framework. Allow the patient to define their own relationships.	*Are you currently involved in any sexual relationships?* *Are you and your partners on the same page about what's pleasurable?*
	Past History of STIs	It is important to refrain from exacerbating feelings of guilt and shame in your patients because they may be already experiencing these feelings and there is no need to add fuel to the fire. An attitude that is negative and risk-based might make it even more difficult for individuals to discuss the topic or to participate in sexual activities that bring them pleasure.	*Have you tested positive for a STI in the past?* *If yes, do you remember what it was? Where was it?* *How was it treated?*
	Protection from STIs	Clinicians should determine the appropriate level of sexual health counseling for each patient, but they also need to acknowledge their own bias and minimizing assumptions based on patient's sexual orientation, gender identity, or relationship framework. Ask about sexual health practices to strike a balance between addressing the unwanted consequences of sex and enjoyment of the sexual relationship.	*Do you and your partners talk openly about sexual desires and boundaries?* *Do you and your partner have a relationship agreement?* *If you use prevention tools (ie, PEP, PrEP, HIV/STI testing, condoms), what methods do you enjoy using the most?* *Are there some kinds of sex where you do not use barriers methods (*that is, *internal and/or external condoms? Why?*
	Practices	Ask open-ended questions about the patient's sexual practices that are focused on the information you need to know based on what you already know about the patient. You can decide where to take the conversation based on the responses.	*Are you able to advocate for sexual pleasure in your relationships?* *Do you use toys (dildos or vibrators) inside your [insert preferred language for genitals] or anus, or do you use them on your partners?* *Which behaviors might expose you to your partners' fluids?*
	Pregnancy Intention	All patients at reproductive age should be asked about their intentions to conceive regardless of their sexual orientation or gender identity. Gender-inclusive language should be used throughout the discussion.	*Are you actively trying to conceive, or do you think that you may conceive at some point within the next year?* *Have you considered using a surrogate?* *What are you and your partner(s) doing to prevent pregnancy?*

Plus	Pleasure	The discussion should include two important elements: events (eg, key features of a sexual occasion, such as the repertoire, timing, and spacing of different sexual practices, occurrence of orgasm, use of a condom or contraception) and people (eg, interactional elements of sexual pleasure, which encompass interpersonal dynamics such as communication, negotiation, and trust).	*How is your sex life?* *Is the sex you're having pleasurable for you? If no, why not?* *Anything else you feel to be important that we did not address?*
	Pride	The discussion should recognize and honor someone's sexual and gender identity from an intersectional perspective (eg, historical context, cultural, structural). Providers and staff should use chosen names, pronouns, and body parts, and respect their patients' partnering decisions.	*What are your pronouns?* *When referring to your genitals, are there specific terms that you use?* *Are you currently on hormone therapy? Have you had any gender-confirming surgeries or procedures?* *What support, if any, do you have from your family and friends about your gender identity and/or sexual orientation?*
	Problems	The discussion should address difficulties related to sex (eg, pain, discomfort, vaginal dryness, lack of arousal, lack of orgasm, lack of erection, low or high level of interest in having sex, mismatched sex drives) as well as sexual violence.	*What concerns do you have about your sex life?* *Are you having any difficulties when you have sex (eg, pain, discomfort, vaginal dryness, lack of arousal, lack of orgasm, and lack of erection)?* *Do you feel safe in your current relationship?* *Are you engaging in sex for pleasure or has anyone ever forced or compelled you do anything sexually that you did not want to do?*

Clinicians should take an inclusive, comprehensive routine sexual history with all patients and be proactive about sexual health, not only problem-focused sexual health appointments by using pleasure positive messaging to communicate effectively and positively. For example, when taking a sexual history using a pleasure-based approach, the "6Ps" technique offers for a complete and inclusive foundation for discussion. This is an extension of the traditional recommendation for sexual history taking by adding the “plus” as the sixth “P,” which includes Pride, Pleasure, and Problems (**Table 3**[36] and Cherabie and colleagues in this issue for additional details on best practices in sexual history taking).

SUMMARY

Sex-positive health care is an essential component in the effort not only to prevent and manage STIs but also to achieve health equity. It has the potential to save lives and enhance community and individual health by providing scientifically grounded information within the context of the pleasure and shifting the burden of addressing health inequities from individuals to organizations and systems. It is essential for providers to acknowledge that patients are consistently learning about themselves and their bodies, navigating the health care system, and developing healthy intimate relationships in a rapidly changing social and political landscape. Clinicians must consistently assess whether the messages conveyed to patients align with either a risk-based or pleasure-based approach. Sex-positive providers ask questions that are open and inclusive without contributing to shame, hold space for experiences that go beyond our societal gender binary, use language that is appropriate for their patients, and remain aware of potential barriers. Sex positivity is a framework that promotes individual preferences while rejecting the traditional taboo of discussing sex, specifically sexual pleasure. It doesn’t matter if someone has multiple sexual partners or if they prefer to be celibate; sex positivity counteracts STI-related stigma and encourages safer sex practices and engagement in care. As a result, sex-positive health practitioners are uniquely positioned to address their demand for holistic services and care that consider their experiences and prioritize health equity.

We need more evidence on the integration of sexual pleasure into STI prevention, sexual health-related education, promotion, policies, programs, and services. It is important to evaluate sex-positive and pleasure-inclusive sexual health care for its impact on a range of outcomes, in different contexts and with a wider range of groups of people, with diverse sexual identities. As new data emerge in the constantly evolving sexual health sector, it is critical to seek professional development opportunities whenever possible to remain inventive and competent for patient care.

CLINICS CARE POINTS

- Healthcare providers have the responsibility to establish an environment that promotes a welcoming environment for patients to openly engage in discussions pertaining to sexuality, without any fear of being subjected to judgment during their clinical interactions.
- Clinicians have the ability to develop an understanding that extends beyond clinical symptoms, signs, and pathophysiology of ailments to address the obstacles posed by a patient’s environment, allowing them to make decisions that promote their holistic well-being.
- To ensure successful support in promoting sexual empowerment and satisfaction, it is critical for providers to possess an extensive knowledge of sexuality, including sexual pleasure, and

to be open to learning about common physical and mental challenges encountered by clients belonging to diverse cultural backgrounds, sexual orientations, gender identities, age groups, and individuals with disabilities.

- Clinicians should conduct a comprehensive and inclusive routine sexual history with every patient and employ a proactive approach towards sexual health, transcending problem-focused sexual health consultations through the use of positive and pleasure-based messaging to foster effective and constructive communication.

DISCLOSURE

K.T. Bond has received research funding from Gilead Sciences. K.T. Bond and A.E. Radix are supported by the National Institute of Mental Health of the National Institutes of Health under Award Number R25MH087217.

REFERENCES

1. Pitts RA, Greene RE. Promoting positive sexual health. Am J Publ Health 2020; 110(2):149.
2. World Health Organization. Defining sexual health: report of a technical consultation on sexual health, 28–31 January 2002, Geneva. 2006. https://www.who.int/reproductivehealth/topics/gender_rights/defining_sexual_health.pdf?ua=1.
3. Nimbi FM, Galizia R, Rossi R, et al. The biopsychosocial model and the sex-positive approach: an integrative perspective for sexology and general health care. Sex Res Soc Pol 2021;1–15.
4. The Global Advisory Board for Sexual Health and Wellbeing. (2018). SEXUAL PLEASURE: The forgotten link in sexual and reproductive health and right. Available here: https://www.gab-shw.org/resources/training-toolkit/.
5. Ford JV, Corona-Vargas E, Cruz M, et al. The World Association for Sexual Health's declaration on sexual pleasure: A technical guide. Int J Sex Health 2021;33(4):612–42.
6. Gruskin S, Yadav V, Castellanos-Usigli A, et al. Sexual health, sexual rights and sexual pleasure: meaningfully engaging the perfect triangle. Sexual and Reproductive Health Matters 2019;27(1):29–40.
7. Zaneva M, Philpott A, Singh A, et al. What is the added value of incorporating pleasure in sexual health interventions? A systematic review and meta-analysis. PLoS One 2022;17(2):e0261034.
8. Kontomanolis EN, Michalopoulos S, Gkasdaris G, et al. The social stigma of HIV–AIDS: society's role. In: HIV/AIDS-Research and Palliative Care. UK: Dove Press; 2017. p. 111–8.
9. Ransome Y, Thurber KA, Swen M, et al. Social capital and HIV/AIDS in the United States: Knowledge, gaps, and future directions. SSM-Population Health 2018;5: 73–85.
10. Darby RS, Henniger NE, Harris CR. Reactions to physician-inspired shame and guilt. Basic Appl Soc Psychol 2014;36(1):9–26.
11. Frost DM. Social stigma and its consequences for the socially stigmatized. Social and Personality Psychology Compass 2011;5(11):824–39.
12. Eaton LA, Driffin DD, Kegler C, et al. The role of stigma and medical mistrust in the routine health care engagement of black men who have sex with men. Am J Publ Health 2015;105(2):e75–82.

13. Bond KT, Leblanc NM, Williams P, et al. Race-Based Sexual Stereotypes, Gendered Racism, and Sexual Decision Making Among Young Black Cisgender Women. Health Educ Behav 2021;48(3):295–305.
14. Prather C, Fuller TR, Marshall KJ, et al. The Impact of Racism on the Sexual and Reproductive Health of African American Women. J Womens Health (Larchmt) 2016;25(7):664–71.
15. Bond KT, Gunn A, Williams P, et al. Using an Intersectional Framework to Understand the Challenges of Adopting Pre-exposure Prophylaxis (PrEP) Among Young Adult Black Women. Sex Res Soc Pol 2022;19(1):180–93.
16. Agénor M, Zubizarreta D, Geffen S, et al. "Making a Way Out of No Way:" Understanding the Sexual and Reproductive Health Care Experiences of Transmasculine Young Adults of Color in the United States. Qual Health Res 2022;32(1): 121–34.
17. Singer RB, Johnson AK, Crooks N, et al. "Feeling Safe, Feeling Seen, Feeling Free": Combating stigma and creating culturally safe care for sex workers in Chicago. PLoS One 2021;16(6):e0253749.
18. Saadat M, Keramat A, Jahanfar S, et al. Barriers and Facilitators to Accessing Sexual and Reproductive Health Services Among Transgender People: A Meta-Synthesis. Int J Soc Determinants Health Health Serv 2023. https://doi.org/10.1177/27551938231187863. 27551938231187863.
19. Sawicki DA, Meffert BN, Read K, et al. Culturally Competent Health Care for Sex Workers: An Examination of Myths That Stigmatize Sex-Work and Hinder Access to Care. Sex Relatsh Ther 2019;34(3):355–71.
20. Stowell M, Hall A, Warwick S, et al. Promoting sexual health in older adults: Findings from two rapid reviews. Maturitas 2023;177:107795.
21. Virani SS, Alonso A, Aparicio HJ, et al. Heart disease and stroke statistics-2021 update: a report from the American Heart Association. Circulation 2021;143(8). CIR0000000000000950.
22. Yin J, Rämgard M, Wangel AM. Sexual health in diabetes care is a 'hot topic'-A qualitative study with Diabetes Specialist Nurses. J Clin Nurs 2023. https://doi.org/10.1111/jocn.16832.
23. Chowdhury EK, Berk M, Nelson MR, et al. Association of depression with mortality in an elderly treated hypertensive population. Int Psychogeriatr 2019;31(3): 371–81.
24. Peppa M, Manta A. Sexual Dysfunction in Diabetic Patients: he Role of Advanced Glycation End Products. Curr Diabetes Rev 2023. https://doi.org/10.2174/1573399819666230407095522.
25. Marks S. A clinical review of antidepressants, their sexual side-effects, post-SSRI sexual dysfunction, and serotonin syndrome. Br J Nurs 2023;32(14):678–82.
26. Smith S, Kloss JD, Kniele K, et al. Drugs that cause sexual dysfunction. Psychiatry 2007;6(3):111–4.
27. Serretti A, Chiesa A. Treatment-emergent sexual dysfunction related to antidepressants: a meta-analysis. J Clin Psychopharmacol 2009;29(3):259–66.
28. Shiri R, Koskimäki J, Tammela TL, et al. Bidirectional relationship between depression and erectile dysfunction. J Urol 2007;177(2):669–73.
29. Downey MM, Gómez AM. Structural Competency and Reproductive Health. AMA J Ethics 2018;20(3):211–23.
30. Mitchell KR, Lewis R, O'Sullivan LF, et al. What is sexual wellbeing and why does it matter for public health? [published correction appears in Lancet Public Health. 2023 Mar;8(3):e172]. Lancet Public Health 2021;6(8):e608–13.

31. Kizilay F, Gali HE, Serefoglu EC. Diabetes and Sexuality. Sexual Medicine Reviews 2017;5(1):45–51.
32. Federation I.P.P., putting sexuality back into comprehensive sexuality education: making the case for a rights-based, sex-positive approach, 2016, International Planned Parenthood Federation; UK, 2021.
33. Metzl JM, Hansen H. Structural competency: theorizing a new medical engagement with stigma and inequality. Soc Sci Med 2014;103:126–33.
34. Ard KL, MacDonald-Ly A, Demidont AC. Sexual Health Care for Transgender and Gender Diverse People. Medical Clinics 2023;108(2).
35. Cherabie J., Donald Hong D., Reno H.E., Taking a Sexual History: Best Practices. Medical Clinics 2023;108(2).
36. Altarum Institute. Sexual Health and Your Patients: A Provider's Guide. Washington, DC: Altarum Institute; 2016. Updated 2022.

Taking a Sexual History

Best Practices

Donald Hong, MD*, Joseph Cherabie, MD, MSc,
Hilary E. Reno, MD, PhD

KEYWORDS

- Sexual health • History taking • Trauma informed • Culturally aware

KEY POINTS

- Taking a sexual history should fit within a holistic view of sexual health care.
- A sexual history will improve care by focusing on well-being and factors that contribute to sexual health.
- Changing the paradigm from a disease centered model to focusing more on patients and their sexual health goals can only help to decrease stigma, discrimination, shame, and trauma inflicted by the health-care systems on our patients.

INTRODUCTION

Sexually transmitted infections (STIs) are at historically high levels in the United States. Most recent STI surveillance data released by the Centers for Disease Control (CDC) in 2021 continue to show this trend. More than 2.5 million cases of gonorrhea, chlamydia, and syphilis were reported in the United States in 2021. This includes 1.6 million cases of chlamydia, 700,000 cases of gonorrhea, and 180,000 cases of syphilis. Of particular concern is the steady increase in congenital syphilis cases since 2013, with a 219.3% increase in cases since 2017.[1]

Before delving into the best practices in sexual health history taking, it is important to define sexual health. Sexual health, as defined by the World Health Organization, encompasses not only the absence of disease or infirmity but also a state of physical, emotional, mental, and social well-being in relation to sexuality. It involves the ability to have pleasurable and safe sexual experiences, free from coercion, discrimination, and violence.[2] The American Sexual Health Association (ASHA) defines sexual health as "the ability to embrace and enjoy our sexuality throughout our lives. It is an important part of our physical and emotional health."[3] The ASHA definition goes further and describes what being sexually healthy means specifically including the following:

Department of Medicine, Division of Infectious Diseases, Washington University in St. Louis School of Medicine, St. Louis, MO, USA
* Corresponding author. Infectious Diseases Division, Washington University School of Medicine, 4523 Clayton Avenue, Mail Stop Code 8051-043-0015, St. Louis, MO 63110.
E-mail address: dlhong@wustl.edu

Med Clin N Am 108 (2024) 257–266
https://doi.org/10.1016/j.mcna.2023.09.004

- Understanding that sexuality is a natural part of life and involves more than sexual behavior.
- Recognizing and respecting the sexual rights we all share.
- Having access to sexual health information, education, and care.
- Making an effort to prevent unintended pregnancies and sexually transmitted diseases (STDs) and seek care and treatment when needed.
- Being able to experience sexual pleasure, satisfaction, and intimacy when desired.
- Being able to communicate about sexual health with others including sexual partners and healthcare providers."

Recognizing these holistic definitions of sexual health (See Bond and colleagues[4] article in this issue for additional details), health-care providers must approach sexual health history taking with sensitivity, inclusivity, and a trauma-informed perspective.

Many versions of what a sexual history should look like exist[3,5,6] but certain principles are commonly found. Education of health-care providers on sexual history taking can involve reviewing the components of the sexual history but should also include the importance of using nonstigmatizing language, having a patient-centered approach,[5] and practicing trauma-informed and culturally sensitive care.

IMPORTANT COMPONENTS OF SEXUAL HISTORY TAKING

Trauma-informed care is an approach that recognizes the high prevalence of abuse and violence and their potential impact on individuals' physical and mental health. It aims to create a safe and supportive environment that promotes healing and empowerment. This approach is especially crucial for individuals who have experienced sexual trauma/violence, as well as members of marginalized communities, including Black, Indigenous, and People of Color (BIPOC) and sexual and gender minority individuals. Adopting trauma-informed care principles, such as safety, transparency, and empowerment helps health-care providers address the specific needs and experiences of these populations, ensuring their voices are heard, their boundaries respected, and their unique cultural contexts considered.[7] The CDC and National Alliance of State and Territorial AIDS Directors (NASTAD) are 2 organizations that provide resources expanding on the important principles of trauma-informed care.[8,9]

Cultural humility is another essential aspect of providing inclusive sexual health care. Often in medicine, trainings and education have revolved around the concept of cultural competency. Culture competency promotes the idea that a provider can become "competent" in understanding a culture different from their own. However, this assumption of competency suggests that every culture has a defined set of beliefs/ideas that are unlikely to change or evolve over time leading to developments of further stigmatizing stereotypes. It also ignores the intersectionality of individual patients who likely have multiple characteristics (race, gender, sexual orientation, and so forth) that contribute to their ideas and beliefs, and providers are unlikely to be able to determine which are contributing to each individual encounter. In contrast to competency, cultural humility involves acknowledging and challenging one's own cultural biases and actively engaging in self-reflection to promote equitable care. Cultural humility recognizes that health-care providers do not possess comprehensive knowledge of every cultural background or identity and encourages ongoing learning, collaboration, and respect for the patient's values, beliefs, and experiences. It allows providers to admit that they do not know everything about a patient's full cultural background and allows them to learn from patient experiences while also understanding how provider beliefs contribute to each encounter as well. Humility allows for a balance of power between patient and provider, leading to a more open communication. By embracing cultural humility, health-care providers can establish trust, foster effective communication, continuously evaluate themselves and their biases, and deliver patient-centered care that respects the diverse needs and perspectives of individuals seeking sexual health services.[10,11]

Finally, *sex positive care* is an approach that promotes a healthy and affirming attitude toward sexuality (See Bond and colleagues23 in this issue for more details). It emphasizes the importance of understanding and embracing sexuality as a natural and positive aspect of human life. Sex positivity challenges societal norms and stigmas surrounding sex, aiming to foster an environment where individuals feel empowered, comfortable, and free from judgment in expressing their sexuality. Sex positivity recognizes that sexual experiences and expressions can vary widely among individuals, encompassing diverse orientations, identities, preferences, and practices. It embraces the principles of consent, respect, pleasure, and open communication, emphasizing that all consensual and safe sexual experiences, as long as they involve informed participation, are valid and worthy of respect. The concept of sex positivity encourages the dismantling of shame, guilt, and discrimination associated with sexuality. It is important to note that sex positivity does not advocate for irresponsible or harmful behaviors but rather emphasizes informed decision-making, sexual health, and mutual respect.

WHY IS TAKING A SEXUAL HISTORY IMPORTANT?

Taking an adequate sexual health history plays a pivotal role in the prevention, diagnosis, and management of STIs. However, shortcomings in sexual history assessment can result in missed diagnoses, inadequate testing, and suboptimal patient care. The CDC's 2021 STI Treatment Guidelines provide recommendations on primary prevention of STI acquisition by patients, which includes assessment of a patient's likelihood of acquisition by assessing their sexual behaviors. As part of this assessment, a routine sexual history is recommended to determine what STIs a patient may be likely to have acquired, to determine what body sites to test for STIs, and to determine what counseling may help reduce a patient's likelihood of STI acquisition.[10]

However, how often is a sexual health history taken during routine primary care visits, and how comfortable are primary care providers in taking a sexual history? A study by Wimberly and colleagues (2006) showed that 56% of physicians felt adequately trained to take a sexual history, whereas 79% felt comfortable taking sexual histories. Of those surveyed, 58% reported taking a sexual history at routine visits with their patients, with 12% to 34% asking about detailed components of sexual history.[12] A review of Lesbian, gay, bisexual, transgender + (LGBT +) experiences in primary care settings showed that there were frequent barriers to accessing care, need for self-advocacy, care avoidance, and disrespectful communication.[13] Another survey of LGBT + individuals showed high rates of stigma and discrimination including being misgendered, assaulted, and denied health care because of their sexual orientation or gender identity.[14]

In the following sections, we will discuss the potential consequences of inadequate sexual history assessment and outline best practices to guide health-care providers in conducting thorough sexual health history assessments.

Possible Consequences of Inadequate Sexual History Assessment

1. Missed diagnoses of asymptomatic infections: Many STIs, such as gonorrhea and chlamydia, can be asymptomatic, leading to a significant risk of underdiagnosis.

Studies have shown that a substantial proportion of individuals with gonorrhea (55.7%–86.8%) and chlamydia (70.0%–88.8%) report no symptoms at the time of diagnosis.[15] Without proper sexual history assessment, a considerable number of STI cases go undetected, resulting in missed opportunities for timely treatment and potential complications. Although proper sexual history taking can help identify individuals who should be screened for asymptomatic infection, it should be noted that symptomatic STIs can also be missed when a proper sexual history is not obtained. Although a common presentation of urethritis or cervicitis should trigger obtaining a sexual history, routine sexual history taking may be helpful in recognizing less common presentations of STIs. A missed STI diagnosis may lead to improper or inadequate treatment, unnecessary testing, and additional pain and suffering for patients. Lymphogranuloma venereum (LGV), caused by specific serovars of *Chlamydia* can present with rectal pain, bleeding, and even a rectal mass. Multiple case reports describe missed diagnoses of LGV leading to unnecessary testing for inflammatory bowel disease including invasive colonoscopies and biopsies.[16] Diffuse adenopathy that can be seen in acute HIV infection may be worked up initially for lymphoma or other inflammatory conditions, leading both to unnecessary invasive biopsies and to critical delays in starting antiretroviral therapy. Routine sexual history taking allows providers to understand what infections a patient may be at increased likelihood of acquiring, increasing awareness of the possibility of those infections, and allowing them to be considered as part of a full differential diagnosis.

2. Lack of rectal or pharyngeal site testing: Relying solely on urogenital testing for gonorrhea and *Chlamydia* may result in missed diagnoses. These infections can also affect other sites, such as the rectum, pharynx, and conjunctiva. Taking a comprehensive sexual history with accurate data on anatomic exposure sites allows for targeted screening or testing, improving the accuracy of diagnosis and ensuring appropriate treatment. According to one study of patients who reported sexual activity between January 2012 and October 2014, pharyngeal gonorrhea, rectal gonorrhea, and rectal chlamydia rates were 8.5%, 15%, and 16.5%, respectively, among men who have sex with men (MSM) and 3.8%, 4.8%, and 11.8%, respectively, among cisgender women having sex with cisgender men.[17]
3. Pelvic inflammatory disease: Incomplete sexual history assessment may lead to missed opportunities for identifying risk factors and preventing pelvic inflammatory disease (PID). PID is a serious complication of untreated or inadequately treated gonorrhea and *Chlamydia* infections. It can result in chronic pelvic pain, tubal factor infertility, ectopic pregnancy, and other adverse reproductive outcomes. By gathering a thorough sexual history and assessing risk factors, health-care providers can identify individuals with higher likelihood of PID and provide appropriate testing, treatment, and counseling to prevent long-term sequelae.
4. Congenital syphilis: In recent years, there has been a concerning increase in the rates of congenital syphilis, emphasizing the need for robust sexual health history taking and timely testing. Congenital syphilis can lead to serious complications and even death in newborns. Despite the availability of effective interventions, the Centers for Disease Control and Prevention (CDC) reported that a significant proportion of pregnant people with syphilis were not properly diagnosed despite receiving timely care.[18] This highlights the importance of testing for syphilis during pregnancy and, if there are new exposures, testing again for syphilis, reinforcing the need for thorough sexual health history assessment.
5. Stigma/discrimination: Research has shown that sexual and gender minority individuals often experience significant barriers when it comes to receiving comprehensive sexual health care. Studies indicate that sexual and gender minority

populations, including lesbian, gay, bisexual, transgender, and queer (LGBTQ+) individuals, are less likely to have their sexual health needs addressed during medical visits compared with their cisgender heterosexual counterparts. Moreover, this disparity is further exacerbated by high rates of stigma, discrimination, and bias experienced by sexual and gender minority individuals within the health-care system.[6] Negative attitudes, lack of cultural competence, and inadequate provider training contribute to a climate where sexual and gender minority individuals may feel unwelcome or hesitant to disclose their sexual histories or seek appropriate care. Similarly, women and individuals from BIPOC communities may also face similar challenges, including intersecting experiences of gender-based discrimination and racial bias that influence their access to and quality of sexual health-care services. Addressing these disparities requires a commitment to creating inclusive and affirming health-care environments, enhancing provider cultural competency, and promoting awareness of the unique needs and experiences of sexual and gender minority individuals, women, and BIPOC communities (See Ard and colleagues[19] article in this series for additional information on sexual health care for transgender and gender diverse people).

Sexual health history taking goes beyond identifying the likelihood of STIs and includes recognizing the need for patient-centered service delivery involving providers, pharmacy, case management, social work, mental health services that embrace the whole well-being of an individual (Wrap-around service delivery). By gathering a comprehensive sexual health history, health-care providers can identify social determinants of health that influence sexual well-being, such as housing instability, intimate partner violence, substance use, mental health concerns, and access to health-care services. This holistic approach enables the identification of underlying factors that contribute to health disparities and facilitates the provision of appropriate referrals and support services to address patients' comprehensive needs. It also allows for a more patient-centered approach, focusing less on diseases and dysfunction and more on sexual health well-being.

ELEMENTS OF A SEXUAL HISTORY

To ensure comprehensive sexual health history taking, health-care providers should adopt best practices from optimizing the clinical environment to mindfully choosing the language we use to expanding what a sexual history means.

Creating an Inclusive Environment

It is essential to create an inclusive environment for sexual and gender minority persons and individuals who have experienced sexual trauma/violence. Discrimination and stigmatization within health-care settings contribute to health disparities among these populations. Adopting trauma-informed care and cultural humility principles can help health-care providers foster trust, respect, and patient-centered care. This includes creating intake forms that capture necessary information on sex assigned at birth, gender identity, pronouns and name (if different than ID), anatomy, sexual practices, as well as basic demographics. This ensures providers have many of the answers they need to take a thorough sexual history before even seeing the patient.

Importance of Language

Starting the conversation

We must be mindful of the language we use during sexual health history taking, asking, "Is it ok if I ask you some questions about your sexual health?" or "Do you have any concerns about your sexual health today?" These questions put the power in the hands of the patient to lead the conversation in a way that works for them, their cultural background and their past experiences, while also normalizing sexual health history taking.

Avoid risk-based language

This is of the utmost importance to avoid stigma and discrimination. Instead of stating "high-risk sexual practices," consider talking about susceptibility, vulnerability, and likelihood of acquiring STIs. It also helps to avoid moral judgment with respect to how we speak about STIs, so avoid wording such as "unfortunately, you have...". Even saying "Good news, your results came back clear" can insinuate that individuals who have STIs have "bad news" and that they should feel shame. STIs occur and as any other infection or medical condition, shame-based messaging does not make someone more healthy. This is why it best to adopt a people-centered approach as has been used by International AIDS Society in the People First Charter, which emphasizes the use of patient-centered language.[20]

Use terms familiar to the patient and mirror language

It is also important to remember to use terms that are familiar to the patient. For example, for MSM, instead of asking if an individual is the penetrative or receptive anal sexual partner, it may be better to ask if they are top (insertive), bottom (receptive), or versatile (both), which is language that is commonly used within this community to state their sexual preferences and practices. Asking people about their language choices and mirroring language can be a method to build rapport with patients and follows their guidance on how they want their body parts referred to as well as their sexual practices.

Expanding the sexual history

To elaborate further on best practices, let us look at the CDC's Guide to Taking a Sexual History,[6] which updates the 5Ps framework to include the following components of a complete sexual history (See also Table 4 in Bond and colleagues[4] article, in this issue).

1. Partners: Ask what are the gender(s) of your partners? Do your partners have any other sex partners? If inquiring about the number of sexual partners, consider the epidemiologic contact windows for bacterial STIs such as gonorrhea (60 days) and syphilis (90 days or more). Most sources recommend asking about partners in the last 3 or 6 months. There is no evidence to support certain time frames but understanding the number of partners a person has had in the previous 3 months can aid in contact tracing if needed. The goals of these questions are to assess the likelihood of STI exposure and transmission dynamics, including helping with contact tracing in case the patient has STIs.
2. Practices: Ask about specific sexual practices, including vaginal, anal, and oral sex by asking anatomically specific questions. Asking "Do you put your mouth on your partner's genitals such as their penis or vagina?" would reduce confusion about how to define oral sex, for example, ask what the patient defines as sex as people define sex differently. This information assists in guiding diagnostic practices and physical examination, as well as tailoring sexual health goals to the patient and their practices.
3. Protection from STIs: Assess the use of all types of barrier methods, vaccines (eg, human papillomavirus), preexposure prophylaxis (PrEP) for HIV, and PrEP or Post Exposure Prophylaxis for STIs. Discuss how discussing testing with partners can diagnose and treat STIs and reduce transmission. These questions help to open discussion on the many options available to prevent STIs.

4. Past history of STIs: Ask about any history of past STIs, including the type, treatment received, and follow-up. This information helps identify individuals at higher likelihood for recurrent infections because individuals with a history of STIs are having sex within a network where STIs are circulating.
5. Pregnancy intention: Inquire about contraception use and family planning goals to ensure comprehensive reproductive health care and overall sexual health goal setting for individuals of pregnancy potential. Shared decision-making is an important method for supporting patients' choices as well as delivering educational counseling.

There have been proposed expansions to the 5Ps including the following:

Preferences: Expanding on individual's sexual health goals and offering them the education and support they need. An example would be asking, "What does good sex mean to you?" or "What are your sexual health goals?" These allow for the patient to share what their particular sexual preferences and goals are and can be reevaluated during each visit.

Pleasure: Asking patients if they are having pleasurable sex and if not, further discussions about general medical health, sexual functioning, power, consent, violence, and mental health may be explored.[21]

Partner violence: According to the National Intimate Partner and Sexual Violence Survey conducted by the Centers for Disease Control (CDC) and Prevention, approximately 1 in 4 women and 1 in 10 men have experienced some form of physical violence, sexual violence, or stalking by an intimate partner in their lifetime. The same survey found that among women who experienced intimate partner violence (IPV), nearly half (46.7%) reported multiple incidents, indicating that IPV can be a recurring pattern rather than an isolated event. A simple means of asking about IPV is asking, "Do you feel safe in your relationship?" or "Do you have any concerns in your relationship?" For more resources on what to do if a patient reports intimate partner violence, the CDC has more information that can be found here: https://www.cdc.gov/violence prevention/intimatepartnerviolence/index.html.

Pride: Supporting patients in taking pride in their gender identity and sexual orientation, through creating a gender inclusive space with sex positive messaging and language used throughout the visit. Use of pronoun pins and stickers, creating space for individuals to use names other than their legal names, and acknowledging the diversity in sexual practices and expression all are a part of pride (**Table 1**).

There may be options to supplement in-person sexual history taking to provide STI/HIV screening. For people with a trauma history, answering questions about sex may

Table 1
Suggested language shifts to be more gender inclusive, trauma informed, and sex positive

Instead of This	Say This
"Hello, I'm Doctor X."	"Hi, I'm Doctor X. I use he/him pronouns."
"Hey Guys!"	"Hey, (folks, y'all, people, everyone)!"
"Do you know how you can prevent STI's?"	"Let's talk about your sexual health goals."
"Why aren't you using protection?"	"It's ok to have condomless sex. Are there times when you would like to try to use condoms more often?"
"Now I'm going to"	"Is It ok if I?"
"What's wrong (with you)"	"What happened (to you)"
"Good news," "Test results are good," "Everything came back clean"	"You do not have *chlamydia* in your *penis*."

be uncomfortable or cause them stress. Offering a list of STI/HIV testing options may be more comfortable for them. Another consideration is for automated sexual history taking. Answering questions on a tablet computer might be more comfortable for people if the questions are patient-centered and use inclusive language. Examining best practices to increase STI testing in clinics caring for people living with HIV, one study noted the high acceptability of automated STI screening/history taking (93.5%).[22] Automated sexual history likely has a place in sexual health care although nuance, sharing of qualitative information, and discussion are not possible.

Another consideration is for universal screening. Why not perform universal screening for everyone regardless of their sexual history? That may seem as an attractive option, especially when considering increasing rates of STIs or need for HIV testing. However, we need to remember, sexual health is more than just the absence of STIs and HIV. Taking a sexual history helps to inform health practitioners about the general health and well-being of an individual with respect to their sexual health, as well as the need for wrap around services.

SUMMARY

Sexual health history taking is a skill that comes with training, repetition, and normalization; unfortunately, sexual health histories are often incomplete,[23] likely not meeting patients' needs. The AAMC provides recommendations on including sexual health history taking within medical school curricula; however, implementation of such recommendations may be institution specific. Universal principles of respect, making sure individuals feel comfortable sharing intimate details about their sex lives with their health-care providers and recognizing that many individuals may have experienced trauma, stigma, discrimination, and sexual violence, all related to their sexual health and well-being are important. Being aware of these principles and acting accordingly can help make sexual health history more inclusive and welcoming. Furthermore, changing the paradigm from a disease-centered model to focusing more on patients and their sexual health goals can only help to decrease stigma, discrimination, shame, and trauma inflicted by the health-care systems on our patients. It starts and stops with opening the conversation with our patients, understanding that sexual health is not merely the absence of disease, and respecting differences in sexual practices while supporting the sexual health goals of each individual and working toward them.

CLINICS CARE POINTS

- Sexual history is an essential part of any primary care visit and examination. Without proper sexual history, we continue to place our patients at risk for systemic complications of undiagnosed infections, continued community spread of STIs, and continued propagation of the stigma and discrimination that leads many of our sexual and gender minority patients to avoid the medical care they deserve.
- A sexual health visit starts as soon as our patients enter the office. Setting an inclusive, comfortable environment allows providers to begin building the necessary trusting relationship that is needed for a true open conversation.
- The 5Ps of a sexual history provided by the CDC (along with the proposed additional Ps) provide a framework for providers of pertinent information that should be included in every comprehensive sexual health assessment. Providing these questions through a sex-positive, gender-neutral, trauma-informed lens allows all patients to feel supported and included.

DISCLOSURE

D. Hong has no financial disclosures. J. Cherabie has no financial disclosures. H. E. Reno reports grant funding to Washington University from Hologic, United States.

REFERENCES

1. Weinstock HS, Kreisel KM, Spicknall IH, et al. STI Prevalence, Incidence, and Costs in the United States: New Estimates, New Approach. Sex Transm Dis 2021;48(4):207.
2. WHO 2002 - http://www.who.int/reproductivehealth/topics/gender_rights/sexual_health/en.
3. Available at: Home - American Sexual Health Association (ashasexualhealth.org).
4. Bond KT, Radix A. Sexual Health and Wellbeing: a framework to guide care. Medical Clinics 2024;108(2).
5. Stanley E. Althof, Raymond C. Rosen, Michael A. Perelman, and Eusebio Rubio-Aurioles. Standard Operating Procedures for Taking a Sexual History.
6. CDC Guide to Taking a Sexual History https://www.cdc.gov/std/treatment/sexualhistory.pdf.
7. Substance Abuse and Mental Health Services Administration (SAMHSA). (2014). SAMHSA's Concept of Trauma and Guidance for a Trauma-Informed Approach. HHS Publication No. (SMA) 14-4884. Rockville, MD: Substance Abuse and Mental Health Services Administration. Link: https://store.samhsa.gov/product/SAMHSA-s-Concept-of-Trauma-and-Guidance-for-a-Trauma-Informed-Approach/sma14-4884.
8. Infographic. 6 guiding principles to a trauma-informed approach. Centers for Disease Control and Prevention, Centers for Disease Control and Prevention; 2020. www.cdc.gov/orr/infographics/6_principles_trauma_info.htm.
9. Trauma-Informed Approaches Toolkit." NASTAD, nastad.org/trauma-informed-approaches-toolkit. Accessed 22 Sept. 2023.
10. Tervalon M, Murray-García J. Cultural Humility Versus Cultural Competence: A Critical Distinction in Defining Physician Training Outcomes in Multicultural Education. J Health Care Poor Underserved 1998;9(2):117–25. Available at:.
11. Lekas HM, Pahl K, Fuller Lewis C. Rethinking Cultural Competence: Shifting to Cultural Humility. Health Serv Insights 2020 Dec 20;13. https://doi.org/10.1177/1178632920970580. 1178632920970580.
12. Wimberly YH, Hogben M, Moore-Ruffin J, et al. Sexual history-taking among primary care physicians. J Natl Med Assoc 2006;98(12):1924–9.
13. Campbell J, Nathoo A, Chard S, et al. Lesbian, gay, bisexual, transgender and or queer patient experiences in Canadian primary care and emergency departments: a literature review. Cult Health Sex 2023;1–18. https://doi.org/10.1080/13691058.2023.2176548.
14. "Discrimination prevents LGBTQ people from accessing health care." Center for American Progress, 2022, Available at: www.americanprogress.org/article/discrimination-prevents-lgbtq-people-accessing-health-care/.
15. Detels R, Green AM, Klausner JD, et al. The incidence and correlates of symptomatic and asymptomatic Chlamydia trachomatis and Neisseria gonorrhoeae infections in selected populations in five countries. Sex Transm Dis 2011;38(6):503–9.
16. Levy I, Gefen-Halevi S, Nissan I, et al. Delayed diagnosis of colorectal sexually transmitted diseases due to their resemblance to inflammatory bowel diseases. Int J Infect Dis 2018;75:34–8.

17. Bamberger DM, Graham G, Dennis L, et al. Extragenital Gonorrhea and Chlamydia Among Men and Women According to Type of Sexual Exposure. Sex Transm Dis 2019;46(5):329–34.
18. Centers for Disease Control and Prevention. Sexually Transmitted Disease Surveillance 2021. Atlanta: US Department of Health and Human Services; 2023.
19. Ard KL, MacDonald-Ly A, Demidont AC. Sexual Health Care for Transgender and Gender Diverse People. Medical Clinics 2023;108(2).
20. Waters L, Hodson M, Josh J. Language matters: The importance of person-first language and an introduction to the People First Charter. HIV Med 2023;24:3–5.
21. Laura Hinkle B, Candice Joy M. In: Office-Based Approaches to Improve Sexual Health Office-Based STI Management: A Practical Approach to Sexual History Taking and Syndromic Management of Sexually Transmitted Infections", In: Bachmann L., *Sexually transmitted infections in HIV-infected adults and special populations*, A Clinical Guide. Cham, Switzerland: Springer International Publishing; 2017. p. 3–37.
22. Nelson JA, Zha P, Halawani M, et al. Evidence-Based Interventions Implemented into HIV Primary Care Clinics to Make Sexually Transmitted Infection Screening and Testing Routine: Outcomes of a Multi-Site Study. AIDS Patient Care STDS 2022;36(S2):92–103.
23. Brookmeyer KA, Coor A, Kachur RE, et al. Sexual History Taking in Clinical Settings: A Narrative Review. Sex Transm Dis 2021;48(6):393–402.

A Practical Approach to Sexually Transmitted Infection Screening for the Primary Care Clinician

Kevin L. Ard, MD, MPH[a,*], Kenneth H. Mayer, MD[b]

KEYWORDS

• Sexually transmitted infection • Gonorrhea • Chlamydia • Syphilis • Screening
• Sexual health

KEY POINTS

- Sexually transmitted infections (STIs) are common and often asymptomatic but may cause complications without diagnosis and treatment.
- Routine screening for chlamydia, gonorrhea, syphilis, and HIV among sexually active persons is recommended to promote early detection and treatment of these conditions.
- Whether to screen for each condition and how often depends on the patient's sexual history, anatomy, and the presence of factors that increase the likelihood or the potential consequences of STIs (eg, pregnancy).

A 23-year-old non-pregnant, cisgender woman presents to establish primary care. She is asymptomatic and has no known chronic medical problems. She has an intrauterine device. She has had oral and vaginal sex with two cisgender men in the past six months, using condoms approximately half the time.

What, if any, screening tests for sexually transmitted infections (STIs) should she be offered? How would recommendations differ if the patient were a cisgender man who has had oral and insertive and receptive anal sex with two cisgender men in the past six months, or a cisgender man who has had oral and vaginal sex with two cisgender women?

[a] Division of Infectious Diseases, Massachusetts General Hospital, Harvard Medical School, 55 Fruit Street, Boston, MA 02114, USA; [b] Division of Infectious Diseases, The Fenway Institute, Fenway Health, Harvard Medical School, Beth Israel Deaconess Medical Center, 1340 Boylston Street, Boston, MA 02215, USA
* Corresponding author.
E-mail address: Kard@mgh.harvard.edu

Med Clin N Am 108 (2024) 267–278
https://doi.org/10.1016/j.mcna.2023.08.014
medical.theclinics.com

INTRODUCTION

Patients like these are commonly encountered in primary care. Sexually transmitted infections (STIs) are also common, with the Centers for Disease Control and Prevention (CDC) estimating that approximately one in five people in the United States recently had an STI.[1] Various organizations, including CDC, the US Preventive Services Task Force (USPSTF), and local health departments, have issued guidelines on STI screening.[2–4] Their recommendations vary based on the STI in question; the patient's age, anatomy, and the gender of sex partners; the presence of other conditions such as pregnancy or HIV; and the local epidemiology of STIs (eg, the patient's sexual networks). Although evidence-based, these guidelines can be difficult to implement in clinical practice because of the numerous and interrelated factors stipulating which STIs should be screened for and how often. Here, we outline the rationale for STI screening and its potential harms, summarize CDC and USPSTF screening guidelines, and propose a practical screening strategy that can be implemented in primary care. Throughout, we focus on screening for asymptomatic people. For the evaluation of people with STI syndromes or who have known exposure to an STI, please refer to CDC STI treatment guidelines (www.cdc.gov/std/treatment-guidelines)[2] and the relevant sections of this edition of the journal. We focus on chlamydia, gonorrhea, syphilis, trichomoniasis, and also mention HIV; infections such as human papillomavirus, hepatitis B, and hepatitis C may be sexually transmitted, but guidelines on screening for these infections are outside the scope of this article.

WHY SCREEN FOR SEXUALLY TRANSMITTED INFECTIONS?

Screening (ie, testing an asymptomatic individual) is a core aspect of primary care, with primary care clinicians routinely assessing for diabetes mellitus, hypertension, hyperlipidemia, and other conditions. In general, screening is warranted for conditions with an asymptomatic phase when the benefits of screening (eg, preemptive treatment that reduces the likelihood of future negative outcomes) outweigh the potential harms. Multiple STIs—including gonorrhea, chlamydia, and syphilis—can be asymptomatic and persistent and are thus amenable to screening. Several benefits for STI screening have been proposed.

- *Screening and subsequent treatment may prevent the development of STI complications.* This rationale underlies the recommendation to screen for gonorrhea and chlamydia more clearly among cisgender women than cisgender men, because cisgender women are at risk for pelvic inflammatory disease and infertility from these infections, whereas clinical sequelae are less common, and generally less morbid, for cisgender men.[3] This rationale also forms the basis for the recommendation for syphilis screening in pregnancy,[4] because congenital syphilis may have devastating consequences for a fetus or newborn, and for syphilis screening in people living with HIV, who may be more likely to develop neurosyphilis.
- *Screening and subsequent treatment may interrupt STI transmission, contributing to STI control.* Studies demonstrating the impact of STI screening on population-level transmission are rare, but a modeling study of gonorrhea and chlamydia screening among men who have sex with men (MSM) taking HIV pre-exposure prophylaxis (PrEP) suggested that even with declines in condom use, biannual screening would decrease the burden of chlamydia and gonorrhea by approximately 40% over 10 years.[5]
- *Screening and treatment may impede HIV transmission.* STIs facilitate HIV transmission.[6] That said, studies of mass STI treatment have not consistently shown a

reduction in HIV transmission with STI treatment,[7,8] and this rationale for STI screening may be less applicable in the era of biomedical HIV prevention, as PrEP or treatment as prevention (ie, the elimination of sexual transmission of HIV when a person with HIV is taking antiretroviral therapy that consistently suppresses the virus) have shown efficacy despite high STI rates.[9]

- *STIs may indicate risk for HIV and thus confer an indication for PrEP.* Syphilis, for example, is closely linked epidemiologically with HIV incidence,[10] and the presence of a recent syphilis infection is considered an indication for PrEP in CDC guidance.[11] The same is true for gonorrhea, whereas chlamydia is considered an indication for PrEP only among MSM.[11]

WHAT ARE POTENTIAL HARMS OF SCREENING FOR SEXUALLY TRANSMITTED INFECTIONS?

Harms of STI screening may include cost, anxiety on the part of patients, interpersonal and relationship disruption from revelation of an STI diagnosis, and adverse effects of STI treatment. Some experts have also raised concerns that treatment of asymptomatic STIs among people who are unlikely to face long-term health consequences (eg, chlamydia among MSM) may contribute antibiotic overuse and the development of antimicrobial resistance.[12] However, how to weigh the individual and population-level impacts of antimicrobial resistance against the personal and public health benefits of STI screening is unclear.

GUIDELINES

CDC and the USPSTF have both published guidelines for STI screening.[2–4] Similarities include a recommendation for gonorrhea and chlamydia screening in women who are 24 years old or younger, specific recommendations for pregnant people, and more frequent or intensive screening for sexually active MSM. However, the guidelines also differ in their recommendations for men, screening intervals, and the STIs for which they make recommendations. Although the CDC guidelines include transgender and gender diverse people as a separate category, guidance both from CDC and the USPSTF is primarily focused on "men" or "women." These distinctions are best understood as reflecting anatomy; for example, any person younger than 24 years with a cervix would have an indication for gonorrhea and chlamydia screening. This is addressed in further detail in the Approach section below. **Table 1** summarizes and compares CDC and USPSTF screening guidance for a subset of common STIs: chlamydia, gonorrhea, syphilis, and trichomoniasis.[2–4] In several instances, guidelines recommend basing the decision to screen or the frequency of screening on an assessment of STI risk. This is defined variably for different STIs but may include report of multiple sex partners, a sex partner with concurrent partners or a recent STI, inconsistent condom use, a history of transactional sex or incarceration, drug use, and/or race and ethnicity as well as the local epidemiology of STIs. Recommendations for STI screening are also embedded within the HIV in primary care guidelines published by the HIV Medicine Association and in CDCs PrEP guidelines[11–13]; these may also serve as resources for clinicians caring for people with HIV or taking PrEP.

APPROACH

Here, we propose a practical approach to STI screening that is compatible with CDC and USPTF guidelines, is inclusive of people with diverse sexual orientations and

Table 1
Summary of Centers for Disease Control and Prevention and US Preventive Services Task Force screening recommendations for chlamydia, gonorrhea, syphilis, and trichomoniasis

Sexually Transmitted Infection	CDC Screening Guidelines	USPSTF Screening Guidelines
Chlamydia and gonorrhea[a]	Women[c] • Sexually active women, including pregnant women, under 25 y of age at least annually • Sexually active women 25 y of age and older, including pregnant women, at increased risk • Additional third trimester screening for pregnant women under 25 y of age or older women at increased risk	Women • Sexually active women, including pregnant women, under 25 y of age • Sexually active women 25 y of age and older, including pregnant women, at increased risk
	Men • No recommendation for heterosexual men, though screening may be considered in high-prevalence settings • MSM at sites of contact[b] at least annually, and every 3–6 mo if at increased risk Transgender and gender diverse people • Screen based on anatomy and include extragenital testing[a] based on sexual behavior People with HIV • At first HIV evaluation and at least annually thereafter • Consider more frequent screening if at increased risk	Others • No recommendation to screen other people for chlamydia and gonorrhea
Syphilis	Women • Women at increased risk • All pregnant women at the first prenatal visit, again at 28-wk gestation if at high risk, and again at delivery if at high risk	Women • All pregnant women
	Men • Heterosexual men at increased risk • MSM at least annually and every 3–6 mo if at increased risk Transgender and gender diverse people • At least annually based on risk People with HIV • At first HIV evaluation and at least annually thereafter • Consider more frequent screening if at increased risk	Others • Screen adults and adolescents at increased risk (includes MSM and people with HIV)

(*continued on next page*)

Table 1
(*continued*)

Sexually Transmitted Infection	CDC Screening Guidelines	USPSTF Screening Guidelines
Trichomoniasis	Women[d] • Annually for women with HIV • Consider for women without HIV but at increased risk or in high-prevalence settings	No recommendation to screen for trichomoniasis

[a] All people diagnosed with chlamydia or gonorrhea should be screened again 3 mo after treatment because reinfection is common.[2]
[b] Extragenital testing includes rectal testing for chlamydia and rectal and pharyngeal testing for gonorrhea.
[c] Clinicians may pursue rectal chlamydia screening and pharyngeal and rectal gonorrhea screening through shared decision-making with patients depending on a history of potential exposure at those sites.
[d] All sexually active women diagnosed with trichomonas should be rescreened 3 mo after initial treatment because reinfection is common.[2]

gender identities, and can be readily implemented in clinical practice. When deciding if, how, and how often to screen for STIs, clinicians should consider.

1. The patient's sexual history
2. The patient's anatomy
3. The presence of factors which enhance the likelihood of STIs or their sequelae

The Sexual History

A cornerstone of primary and sexual health care, including STI screening, is eliciting a sexual history. Please refer to the dedicated article in this journal for a detailed discussion about obtaining a sexual history. The process of eliciting the sexual history should be free of judgment and assumptions about sexual practices, anatomy, and the gender and anatomy of sex partners. When deciding about STI screening, key elements to ask about include the number of people with whom the patient had had any sexual contact in a recent timeframe; a reasonable approach is to ask initially about the past 12 months. Clinicians can later adjust the timeframe depending on the frequency of visits and the patient's sexual activity. For example, patients taking PrEP, who are generally seen every 2 to 3 months depending on their PrEP medication,[11] can be asked about sexual activity since the last visit. Establishing the exact number of sexual partners is less important than understanding if the patient has not had sex in that timeframe, has had sex with one person only, or has had sex with more than one person. Understanding the context of sexual activity can also help assess the likelihood of STIs. For example, people who report sexual contact at saunas or bathhouses or those who engage in group sex may have a greater likelihood of STIs than those who report sex outside of these contexts.[14]

A second key element of sexual history taking is to inquire about sexual behaviors and, in particular, sites of anatomic exposure during sex. Extragenital infections with gonorrhea and chlamydia are common,[15] so all patients who report sex should be asked about insertive and receptive oral and anal sex in addition to genital contact. Although it can be helpful to ask about use of condoms or other strategies to prevent pregnancy or STIs, screening should not be deferred if patients report frequent condom use, because protection provided by condoms is imperfect and condoms are uncommonly used for some activities that readily transmit STIs (eg, oral sex).[16,17] CDC guidelines recommend extragenital screening for gonorrhea and chlamydia for MSM and suggest it can be considered based on the sexual history and through shared decision-making for other groups.[2] However, offering extragenital screening more broadly to all people who report oral and/or rectal contact may be warranted. Pharyngeal gonococcal infections, for example, are often asymptomatic but may be an important source of transmission to others.[18] Screening for asymptomatic pharyngeal chlamydia is not recommended because its clinical significance is uncertain and it frequently clears spontaneously.[2]

Although the sexual history is a vital step in sexual health care and STI screening, clinicians may encounter barriers in eliciting the sexual history. Stigma, confidentiality concerns, time pressure, or simply a failure to ask about key aspects of sexual behavior may limit the information available.[19,20] The assessment of likelihood for STIs based on a sexual history also often features uncertainty because information about a sexually-active person's sex partners—for example, whether they have STIs or have concurrent sexual partners—is not known. For these reasons, screening recommendations for chlamydia, gonorrhea, and syphilis suggest that clinicians consider the local epidemiology of STIs (eg, high syphilis prevalence in the community) in decisions to screen, in addition to sexual behaviors reported by patients.[2–4]

The Patient's Anatomy

Like the sexual history, understanding the patient's anatomy is crucial for deciding how to screen for STIs as well as for other aspects of primary care (eg, whether cervical cancer screening is warranted). Although clinicians may be most familiar with considering variations in genital anatomy for transgender, gender diverse, and intersex people, establishing the anatomy that is present is important for all patients. For the purposes of STI screening, the presence or absence of the penis, testicles, vagina, cervix, ovaries, and uterus should be determined. This information, sometimes called an anatomic or organ inventory, can be elicited as part of the visit and recorded in structured fields within the electronic medical record.[21]

The Presence of Factors Which Enhance the Likelihood of Sexually Transmitted Infection or Sequelae from Them

Four additional characteristics or conditions impact STI screening recommendations: the combination of age and anatomy, pregnancy, HIV, and use of PrEP.

Both CDC and USPSTF guidelines recommend chlamydia and gonorrhea screening for women younger than 25 years, because these infections are common among young women and because untreated infections may lead to pelvic inflammatory disease and/or infertility.[2,3] Because the sequelae of chlamydia and gonorrhea relate to anatomy but not gender identity, this recommendation should be implemented for all people with a vagina and cervix who are younger than 25 years.

STIs in pregnancy are associated with adverse outcomes, including preterm birth and postnatal complications in the case of chlamydia and gonorrhea and congenital infection in the case of syphilis, which can be prevented by treatment.[3,4] All pregnant people should be screened for syphilis, HIV, and chlamydia and gonorrhea. In the setting of rising numbers of congenital syphilis cases,[22] clinicians should also carefully follow local public heath recommendations regarding repeat syphilis screening in pregnancy; repeat screening at 28 weeks gestation and at delivery is recommended in areas with high prevalence of syphilis or if at increased risk.[2]

Because STIs and HIV can be acquired through similar mechanisms and because some STIs may have more severe manifestations in those with advanced HIV-associated immunosuppression (eg, syphilis), STI screening is recommended on entry into care for people diagnosed with HIV and subsequently at a frequency determined by the patient's sexual behavior.[2,13] This recommendation can be adjusted based on the sexual history; for example, if a patient with HIV is not sexually active or reports a long-term, mutually monogamous relationship, annual screening for bacterial STIs may not be necessary.

The final additional factor that impacts decisions about STI screening is whether the patient is taking PrEP for HIV. Bacterial STIs are common among people prescribed PrEP; in one cohort of predominantly MSM receiving oral PrEP, half acquired gonorrhea, chlamydia, or syphilis over 1 year.[9] CDC has also published guidance about STI screening among people taking PrEP, with recommendations for every 3 month screening for gonorrhea, chlamydia, and syphilis for MSM and transgender women taking oral PrEP, every 6 month screening for others on oral PrEP, every 4 month screening for MSM and transgender women taking long-acting injectable cabotegravir for PrEP, and every 6 month screening for others taking long-acting injectable cabotegravir.[11] Because STIs are common among MSM who are eligible for PrEP,[23] clinicians can consider offering the same panel and frequency of STI screening tests to MSM without HIV who are not taking PrEP.

What to Screen for and How to Screen

Table 2 shows the preferred screening tests for common STIs. Nucleic acid amplification tests (NAATs) are preferred for diagnosis of chlamydia and gonorrhea because their sensitivity exceeds that of culture.[2] The best specimen type for NAAT depends on the anatomic site. For testing the throat, rectum, endocervix, and vagina, a swab should be obtained.[2,24] The sensitivity of vaginal and endocervical swabs is similar, so collecting an endocervical specimen is not required if a vaginal swab can be obtained. For testing the penile urethra, a first-catch urine sample, a self-collected meatal swab, and a urethral swab are all acceptable specimen types.[2,25,26] Urine testing in people with vaginas is possible but is less sensitive than a vaginal swab.[24] With proper instructions, throat, rectal, and vaginal swabs for NAAT can be self-collected by patients without a decrement in accuracy.[2]

The preferred screening test for syphilis is a serologic assay. Syphilis tests are broadly divided into non-treponemal assays (eg, the rapid plasma regain [RPR]) which are not specific to syphilis but reflect disease activity and treponemal assays (eg, the treponemal antibody), which are more specific for syphilis but do not reflect disease activity and may persist indefinitely.[2] Two screening strategies are commonly used. In the traditional approach, blood is screened with a non-treponemal assay; if this is positive, a treponemal assay is performed for confirmation. Increasingly, however, a reverse algorithm is being used to test for syphilis. In the reverse algorithm, blood is first tested with a treponemal test; if this is positive, a non-treponemal test is performed for confirmation. If the non-treponemal test is negative, a second treponemal

Table 2
Preferred screening tests for common sexually transmitted infections

Infection(s)	Preferred Screening Test
Chlamydia and gonorrhea	Swab for NAAT from the throat, rectum, vagina, or endocervix Urine or meatal swab for NAAT from the penile urethra
Syphilis	Serology
Trichomonas	Swab for NAAT from the vagina or endocervix; urine sample
HIV	Antibody/antigen assay (+ HIV viral assay if recent antiretroviral exposure)

assay, ideally targeting a different antigen, is performed. Clinicians often do not determine whether the traditional or reverse algorithm is used; rather, this is determined by the protocols of the performing laboratory. Because treponemal tests may remain positive for life in people with prior syphilis, assessing for a sustained fourfold increase in non-treponemal assay is necessary to diagnose new infection when screening someone with a history of syphilis (see Gilliams and colleagues in this series for additional details on syphilis serologies).

Of note, as per CDC guidelines, individuals diagnosed with gonorrhea or chlamydia and sexually active women diagnosed with trichomonas should be rescreened 3 months after treatment as reinfection is common. Syphilis serologies are recommended to be followed at intervals after treatment (See Gilliams and colleagues in this series).[2]

CDC guidelines recommend screening for *Trichomonas vaginalis* infection annually in women with HIV and consideration for women in high-prevalence settings or who otherwise face an increased likelihood of trichomoniasis because they have multiple sex partners, engage in transactional sex, use drugs, or are incarcerated.[2] Following an anatomy-focused approach, this recommendation should be extended to all people with a vagina and cervix who have HIV or are otherwise at risk. Although wet mount vaginal microscopy can detect *Trichomonas*, NAAT (which can be done on vaginal, endocervical, and urine specimens) is preferred for screening due to superior sensitivity.[27] Per CDC guidelines, pregnant women who are living with HIV should be screened for *T vaginalis* in the first trimester.

Sex is the most frequent mode of transmission for HIV.[28] CDC and USPSTF guidelines recommend that adults and adolescents are screened for HIV (ages 13–64 years in CDC guidance and 15–65 years in USPSTF guidance) at least once.[2,29] In addition, screening for HIV should be included as a component of STI screening whenever this screening is performed for people not known to have the infection and all pregnant people at the first prenatal visit and in the third trimester if at higher risk. HIV screening is also recommended at least annually for MSM, more often for those at increased likelihood of HIV or who are taking PrEP (ie, every 2–3 months depending on the PrEP modality used). The preferred screening test for HIV is the laboratory-based antibody/antigen serologic assay unless the patient has recently been exposed to antiretrovirals, such as through PrEP or HIV post-exposure prophylaxis (PEP); in those scenarios, an HIV RNA assay should also be included because antiretroviral exposure may delay positivity of the antibody/antigen test.[2,11]

What Not to Screen for

Routine screening is not recommended for *Mycoplasma genitalium* and other *Mycoplasma* species, *Ureaplasma* species, and herpes simplex virus (HSV). Routine screening for *M genitalium* is not currently recommended because the clinical significance of asymptomatic infection is uncertain and because of increasing concerns about antimicrobial resistance if asymptomatic cases are treated.[2] Pregnant women should not be routinely screened for *M genitalium*. However, it is reasonable to screen individuals for *M genitalium* if they have had recent sexual contact with a person with symptomatic, confirmed *M genitalium* infection. The pathogenicity and role of other *Mycoplasma* species and *Ureaplasma* is uncertain, and there are no established benefits to routine screening for these organisms.[30] Although CDC guidance indicates that HSV screening can be considered for people presenting for STI evaluation, the USPTSF recommends against routine serologic screening for HSV, because the test has a substantial false-positive rate.[31] In addition, it is uncertain how to best counsel or treat patients with a positive result, particularly when they have never had symptoms

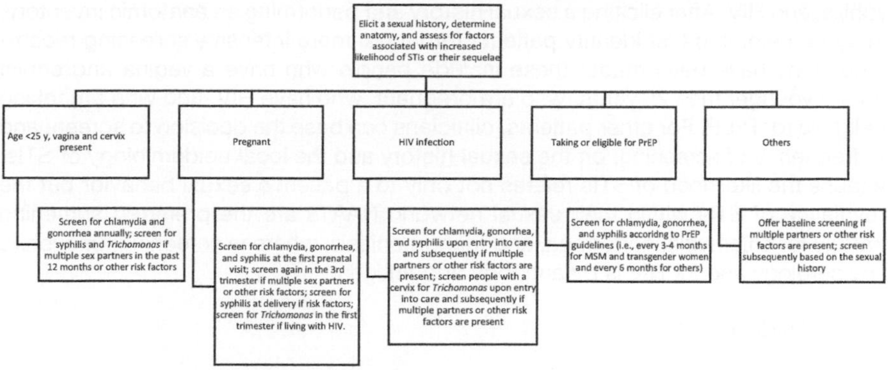

Fig. 1. An approach to STI screening in primary care. HIV screening is recommended every time a person is tested for other STIs, unless they are already known to have HIV.

of HSV. See Batteiger and colleagues and Obafemi and colleagues in this issue for more in depth discussion of HSV and *M genitalium*, respectively.

DISCUSSION: PUTTING SEXUALLY TRANSMITTED INFECTION SCREENING INTO PRACTICE

When considering STI screening, clinicians can follow an approach such as that summarized by the algorithm in **Fig. 1**. After eliciting the sexual history and asking about anatomy, clinicians can first consider if their patient is younger than 25 years with a vagina and cervix, is pregnant, has HIV, or is taking or eligible for PrEP. The rationale for first considering these factors is that they often confer indications for more extensive STI screening than would otherwise be recommended. For these individuals, the frequency of repeat STI screening can be based on the sexual history and local epidemiology of STIs. For other sexually active patients, it is reasonable to offer baseline screening for STIs (for chlamydia, gonorrhea, syphilis, HIV, and *Trichomonas* for those with a vagina and cervix) if risk factors are present (eg, multiple recent sex partners), with the frequency of subsequent screening based on the sexual history.

Clinical vignette follow-up: Applying this approach to the cases at the beginning of this article, the first patient has multiple recent sex partners and is younger than 25 years with a vagina and cervix; she should be offered vaginal NAATs for chlamydia, gonorrhea, and trichomoniasis; pharyngeal NAAT for gonorrhea; and blood testing for HIV and syphilis. The second patient is a cisgender man who has sex with men with multiple recent sex partners who is eligible for PrEP; we would offer him rectal and urine NAATs for chlamydia and gonorrhea, a pharyngeal NAAT for gonorrhea, and blood testing for HIV and syphilis. We would also offer him PrEP and repeat STI screening in 3 months. The third patient is a cisgender man who has sex with women with multiple recent sex partners; we would offer him a urine NAAT for gonorrhea and chlamydia; a pharyngeal NAAT for gonorrhea; and blood testing for HIV and syphilis.

SUMMARY

Rates of STIs are increasing in the United States, and STI screening is a key aspect of preventive care and health promotion for patients in primary care. Clinicians can readily implement CDC and USPSTF STI screening guidelines for chlamydia, gonorrhea, syphilis, and HIV. After eliciting a sexual history and performing an anatomic inventory, it may be helpful to first identify patients for whom more intensive screening recommendations have been made; these include people who have a vagina and cervix and are younger than 25 years, who are pregnant, who have HIV, and who are taking or eligible for PrEP. For other patients, clinicians can base the decision to screen, and the frequency of screening, on the sexual history and the local epidemiology of STIs, because the likelihood of STIs relates not only to a patient's sexual behavior but the prevalence of STIs within their sexual network. NAATs are the preferred screening strategy for chlamydia, gonorrhea, and trichomoniasis, whereas screening for syphilis is by serology and for HIV is by antibody and antigen.

CLINICS CARE POINTS

- Clinical decision-making around sexually transmitted infection (STI) screening relies on the sexual history, understanding patients' anatomy, and considering if there are additional factors which increase the likelihood of STIs or their sequelae. These factors include age less than 25 years with a vagina and cervix present, pregnancy, concurrent HIV, receipt of HIV pre-exposure prophylaxis (PrEP), and contact with partners at higher likelihood of STIs.
- The preferred screening strategy for chlamydia and gonorrhea is the nucleic acid amplification test (NAAT). Samples are obtained via swabs for the pharynx, rectum, vagina, and endocervix. For testing the penile urethra, urine is the preferred specimen type.
- For people with a vagina and cervix who are eligible for trichomoniasis screening, the preferred specimen type is a vaginal or endocervical NAAT.
- Screening for syphilis may begin with a non-treponemal test or a treponemal test, depending on the performing laboratory's protocols. If the initial test is positive, a second test of a different type (eg, treponemal test if the initial test was a non-treponemal test) should be performed for confirmation.
- The optimal screening test for HIV is the antibody/antigen test. HIV RNA testing may be helpful for patients with symptoms compatible with acute HIV infection and/or those using PrEP.
- Screening for herpes simplex virus, *M genitalium* and other *Mycoplasma* species, and *Ureaplasma* species is not recommended.

DISCLOSURE

Dr K.L. Ard has received in-kind research support from Binx Health. Dr K.H. Mayer has received unrestricted research grants from Gilead Sciences, United States, ViiV Healthcare, United Kingdom, and Merck, United States and is on the Scientific Advisory Boards of Gilead Sciences and Merck, Inc related to HIV.

REFERENCES

1. Kreisel KM, Spicknall IH, Gargano JW, et al. Sexually transmitted infections among US women and men: Prevalence and incidence estimates, 2018. Sex Transm Dis 2021;48(4):208–14.
2. Workowski KA, Bachmann LH, Chan PA, et al. Sexually transmitted infections treatment guidelines, 2021. MMWR Recomm Rep (Morb Mortal Wkly Rep) 2021;70(4):1–192.
3. US Preventive Services Task Force, Davidson KW, Barry MJ, et al. Screening for chlamydia and gonorrhea. JAMA 2021;326(10):949–56.

4. US Preventive Services Task Force, Curry SJ, Krist AH, et al. Screening for syphilis infection in pregnant women. JAMA 2018;320(9):911–7.
5. Jenness SM, Weiss KM, Goodreau SM, et al. Incidence of gonorrhea and chlamydia following human immunodeficiency virus preexposure prophylaxis among men who have sex with men: a modeling study. Clin Infect Dis 2017;65(5):712–8.
6. Sexton J, Garnett G, Rottingen JA. Metaanalysis and metaregression in interpreting study variability in the impact of sexually transmitted diseases on susceptibility to HIV infection. Sex Transm Dis 2005;32(6):351–7.
7. Wawer MJ, Sewankambo NK, Serwaddo D, et al. Control of sexually transmitted diseases for AIDS prevention in Uganda: a randomized community trial. Lancet 1999;353(9152):525–35.
8. Hayes RJ, Watson-Jones D, Celum C, et al. Treatment of sexually transmitted infections for HIV prevention: End of the road or new beginning. AIDS 2010; 24(Suppl 4):S15–26.
9. Volk JE, Marcus JL, Phengrasamy T, et al. No new HIV infections with increasing use of HIV preexposure prophylaxis in a clinical practice setting. Clin Infect Dis 2015;61(10):1601–3.
10. Solomon MM, Mayer KH, Glidden DV, et al. Syphilis predicts HIV incidence among men and transgender women who have sex with men in a pre-exposure prophylaxis trial. Clin Infect Dis 2014;59(7):1020–6.
11. Preexposure prophylaxis for the prevention of HIV in the United States – 2021 update. Centers for Disease Control and Prevention. 2021. Accessed 25 Jun 2023. Available at: https://www.cdc.gov/hiv/pdf/risk/prep/cdc-hiv-prep-guidelines-2021.pdf.
12. Kenyon C, Vanbaelen T, van Dijck C. Recent insights suggest the need for the STI field to embrace a more eco-social conceptual framework: a viewpoint. Int J STD AIDS 2022;33(4):404–15.
13. Thompson MA, Horberg MA, Agwu AL, et al. Primary care guidance for persons with human immunodeficiency virus: 2020 update by the HIV Medicine Association of the Infectious Diseases Society of America. Clin Infect Dis 2021;73(11): e3572–605.
14. Buttram ME, Kurtz SP. Frequency of group sex participation and risk for HIV/STI among young adult nightclub scene participants. Int J Sex Health 2018; 30(1):12–9.
15. Chan PA, Robinette A, Montgomery M, et al. Extragenital infections caused by Chlamydia trachomatis and Neisseria gonorrhoeae: a review of the literature. Infect Dis Obstet Gynecol 2016;2016:5758387.
16. Stone N, Hatherall B, Ingham R, et al. Oral sex and condom use among young people in the United Kingdom. Perspect Sex Reprod Health 2006;38(1):6–12.
17. Javanbakht M, Westmoreland D, Gorbach P. Factors associated with pharyngeal gonorrhea in young people: Implications for prevention. Sex Transm Dis 2018; 45(9):588–93.
18. Barbee LA, Khosropour C, Dombrowski JC, et al. An estimate of the proportion of symptomatic gonococcal, chlamydial, and non-gonococcal non-chlamydial urethritis attributable to oral sex among men who have sex with men: a case-control study. Sex Transm Infect 2016;92(2):155–60.
19. Palaiodimos L, Herman HS, Wood E, et al. Practices and barriers in sexual history taking: a cross-sectional study in a public adult primary care clinic. J Sex Med 2020;17:1509–19.
20. Barbee LA, Dhanireddy S, Tat SA, et al. Testing of HIV-infected men who have sex with men engaged in HIV primary care. Sex Transm Dis 2015;42(10):590–4.

21. Grasso C, Goldhammer H, Thompson J, et al. Optimizing gender-affirming medical care through anatomical inventories, clinical decision support, and population health management in electronic health record systems. J Am Med Inform Assoc 2021;28(11):2531–5.
22. Sexually transmitted disease surveillance 2021. Centers for Disease Control and Prevention; 2023. Available at: https://www.cdc.gov/std/statistics/2021/default.htm. Accessed 26 June 2023.
23. Nguyen VK, Greenwald ZR, Trottier H, et al. Incidence of sexually transmitted infections before and after pre-exposure prophylaxis for HIV. AIDS 2018;32(4):523–30.
24. Aaron KJ, Griner S, Footman A, et al. Vaginal swab vs urine for detection of *Chlamydia trachomatis, Neisseria gonorrhoeae*, and *Trichomonas vaginalis*: a meta-analysis. Ann Fam Med 2023;21(2):172–9.
25. Dize L, Barnes P Jr, Barnes M, et al. Performance of self-collected penile-meatal swabs compared to clinician-collected urethral swabs for the detection of Chlamydia trachomatis, Neisseria gonorrhoeae, *Trichomonas vaginalis*, and *Mycoplasma genitalium* by nucleic acid amplification assays. Diagn Microbiol Infect Dis 2016;86(2):131–5.
26. Chernesky MA, Jang D, Portillo E, et al. Self-collected swabs of the urinary meatus diagnose more Chlamydia trachomatis and Neisseria gonorrhoeae infections than first catch urine from men. Sex Transm Infect 2013;89(2):102–4.
27. Muzny CA, Blackburn RJ, Sinsky R, et al. Added benefit of nucleic acid amplification testing for the diagnosis of *Trichomonas vaginalis* among men and women attending a sexually transmitted diseases clinic. Clin Infect Dis 2014;59(6):834–41.
28. Diagnoses of HIV infection in the United States and dependent areas, 2021. HIV Surveillance Report. Centers for Disease Control and Prevention; 2023. Available at: https://www.cdc.gov/hiv/basics/statistics.html. Accessed 3 July 2023.
29. US Preventive Services Task Force, Owens DK, Davidson KW, et al. Screening for HIV infection. JAMA 2019;321(23):2326–36.
30. Horner P, Donders G, Cusini M, et al. Should we be testing for urogenital Mycoplasma hominis, Ureaplasma parvum, and Ureaplasma urealyticum in men and women? – a position statement from the European STI Guidelines Editorial Board. J Eur Acad Dermatol Venereol 2018;32(11):1845–51.
31. US Preventive Services Task Force, Mangione CM, Barry MJ, et al. Serologic screening for genital herpes infection. JAMA 2023;329(6):502–7.

The Management of Gonorrhea in the Era of Emerging Antimicrobial Resistance

What Primary Care Clinicians Should Know

Laura A.S. Quilter, MD, MPH[1,*], Sancta B. St. Cyr, MD, MPH[1],
Lindley A. Barbee, MD, MPH

KEYWORDS

• *Neisseria gonorrhoeae* • Gonorrhea • Sexually transmitted infections
• Antimicrobial resistance

KEY POINTS

- *Neisseria gonorrhoeae*'s ability to develop resistance to antimicrobials remains a challenge.
- Nucleic acid amplification tests are considered the preferred test for the detection of *N. gonorrhoeae*; however, culture is the only modality that allows for comprehensive antimicrobial susceptibility testing.
- The recommended treatment for uncomplicated gonorrhea in adults and adolescents at all anatomic sites is ceftriaxone 500 mg intramuscular once as it is the only remaining highly effective single-dose regimen; thus, a reported beta-lactam allergy should prompt a review to determine whether a true allergy is present.
- Test of cure is recommended for everyone diagnosed with pharyngeal gonorrhea.
- Clinicians should work with local and state partners to manage suspected gonorrhea treatment failure cases.

BACKGROUND

Gonorrhea is caused by *Neisseria gonorrhoeae*, a gram-negative diplococcus. The bacterium, a strictly human pathogen transmitted primarily by sexual contact, causes both symptomatic and asymptomatic infections. Asymptomatic infections can contribute to delays in medical care, onward transmission in a community, and

Division of STD Prevention, Centers of Disease Control and Prevention, 1600 Clifton Road Northeast, MS H24-4, Atlanta, GA 30329, USA
[1] Co-first authors.
* Corresponding author. Division of STD Prevention, Centers of Disease Control and Prevention, 1600 Clifton Road Northeast, MS H24-4, Atlanta, GA 30329.
E-mail address: lquilter@cdc.gov

Med Clin N Am 108 (2024) 279–296
https://doi.org/10.1016/j.mcna.2023.08.015
0025-7125/24/Published by Elsevier Inc.

complications such as pelvic inflammatory disease (PID). Gonorrhea is a public heath challenge, particularly due to the organism's ability to develop antimicrobial resistance. Current control methods rely on prevention, timely diagnosis, and appropriate treatment.

Epidemiology

Gonorrhea is the second most commonly reported bacterial infection in the United States (US) with 710,151 cases reported to the Centers for Disease Control and Prevention (CDC) in 2021.[1] After decades of declining gonorrhea rates, the early 2000s initiated a reverse in trends with continuously increasing rates. However, the true incidence of disease is uncertain due to underdiagnosis and under reporting. It is estimated that 1.6 million incident gonococcal infections occur in the US annually and 82.3 million occur globally.[2,3]

Gonorrhea epidemiology highlights major health disparities in the US, mostly attributed to environmental factors, limited resources, and unequal access to health care.[4] Differences appear by age, gender, geographic region, race, and sexual orientation. Overall, gonorrhea is more common in men than in women and is highest in both men and women aged 20 to 24 years.[1] The US South region and non-Hispanic Black or African American persons have the highest reported case rates. Additionally, test positivity for gonorrhea was highest among gay, bisexual, and other men who have sex with men (MSM) at 22.7%, followed by men who have sex with women only (MSW) at 12.2%, and women at 5.9%.[1]

Antimicrobial Resistance in Gonorrhea

Neisseria gonorrhoeae's ability to develop resistance to antimicrobials has been a persistent challenge since the early 20th century.[5] Sulfonamides were introduced in the late 1930s and by the 1940s resistance to high doses of sulfonamides was widespread. In the 1940s and 1950s, penicillins, aminoglycosides, and macrolides were introduced, with penicillins becoming the preferred treatment. Despite early resistance development, penicillin was able to be used for gonorrhea treatment for over 40 years due to its safety and tolerability allowing gradual increases of curative dosing until the 1980s. Tetracyclines, introduced in the 1960s, were used as an alternative to penicillin until resistance became widespread in the 1980s.

Newer antimicrobials like cephalosporins and fluoroquinolones were introduced in the 1980s. By the 1990s, resistance to fluoroquinolones began to appear and quickly spread across the US in the early 2000s. Third-generation cephalosporins were left as the drugs of choice for gonococcal treatment.[5] Because of signs of developing resistance to cefixime and reported treatment failures in 2010, cefixime was removed as a recommended regimen,[6] and rising rates of azithromycin with elevated minimum inhibitory concentrations (MICs) led to the drugs removal as an alternative treatment in 2015, and as a co-therapy in 2020.[7] Now, ceftriaxone, the injectable third-generation cephalosporin, is the last remaining highly effective single-dose drug available for empiric single-dose gonorrhea treatment. *Neisseria gonorrhoeae*'s constant adaptation to different antimicrobials has required regular updates to national gonorrhea treatment recommendations to maintain effective treatment options.

Clinical Manifestations and Transmission

Neisseria gonorrhoeae initially infects non-cornified epithelium, the mucous membranes, of the urogenital tract, the rectum, the oropharynx, and conjunctivae. In some cases, the organism can cross into the blood stream from these mucosal sites and cause a disseminated infection (**Table 1**).

Urogenital Infection

Gonorrhea is associated with urogenital clinical syndromes including urethritis, epididymitis, cervicitis, and PID. However, a high proportion of persons with urogenital gonorrhea may be asymptomatic; up to 70% of women with cervical infections may not present with symptoms.[8] The relative proportion of urethral infection that remains asymptomatic is somewhat unclear. Clinic-based studies suggest that urethral gonorrhea is primarily a symptomatic infection,[9,10] but some population-based studies estimate that up to 60% of men with urethral gonorrhea may be asymptomatic or present only with mild symptoms.[11,12] Epididymitis is the most common local complication of gonococcal urethritis, though the frequency of urethral infection progression to epididymitis in the modern era of antimicrobial therapy remains unknown.[13] PID has been estimated to occur in 10% to 20% of those with untreated cervical gonorrhea.[14,15]

Rectal Infection

Although rectal gonococcal infections have been associated with receptive anal intercourse, they can be detected in the absence of reported rectal sexual exposure. In a systemic review of extragenital gonorrhea, the prevalence of rectal infection among MSM was estimated to be 6% (median; range 0.2%–24%) compared with 3% (median; range 0%–5.7%) among MSW and 2% (median; range 0.6%–36%) among women.[16] In women, anorectal gonorrhea may be acquired through autoinoculation in the absence of receptive anal intercourse. Among men who report no receptive anal intercourse the route of transmission is unclear, but may be due to analingus.[17] Gonococcal infections at the rectum are typically asymptomatic, though proctitis may occur.[18]

Pharyngeal Infection

The pharynx is a common site of gonococcal infection and is typically asymptomatic. The prevalence of pharyngeal gonorrhea, among MSM, has been found to be greater than 10%, and among women and heterosexual men, 2% to 10%.[16,19] Additionally, among heterosexual contacts to gonorrhea, approximately 20% to 50% test positive at the throat.[20,21] Pharyngeal gonorrhea is thought to be acquired primarily via oral-genital contact, though some literature suggests kissing could be a primary transmission mode.[22]

Conjunctival Infection

Historically, gonococcal conjunctivitis was a disease of infants due to acquisition from untreated mothers during birth; however, it can also occur in adults and adolescents as a result of autoinoculation from an anogenital infection. Person-to-person nonsexual contact, fomites, and vectors have been reported in outbreaks of gonococcal conjunctivitis.[23,24] Gonococcal conjunctivitis in infants (ie, ophthalmia neonatorum) has been a rare event in the modern era due to routine prophylaxis with antibiotic eye ointment application to infants at birth.[25]

Disseminated Gonococcal Infection

Historically, disseminated gonococcal infection (DGI) has been rare, occurring in 0.5% to 3% of untreated gonococcal infections[26]; however, as rates of gonorrhea continue to increase, clinicians may see rare gonococcal clinical presentations more frequently. Clinical manifestations of DGI include skin lesions, tenosynovitis, asymmetric polyarthralgia, septic arthritis, and, on rare occasions, endocarditis, meningitis, or osteomyelitis. Since 2019, DGI clusters and increases in DGI cases have been reported in some US states, Manitoba, Canada, and England.[27–30] Among 274 DGI cases

Table 1
Clinical syndromes and infections caused by *Neisseria gonorrhoeae*

Anatomic Site of Infection	Associated Syndrome	Signs and Symptoms	Complications	Comments
Male urogenital infections				
Urethra	Urethritis	Copious urethral discharge, purulent or mucopurulent in color; dysuria	Periurethral abscesses, penile edema, penile lymphangitis, prostatitis	Discharge may not be distinguishable on examination from the discharge seen in nongonococcal urethritis
Epididymis	Epididymitis	Unilateral testicular pain, testicular swelling, dysuria	Abscess, testicular infarction, decreased fertility	N/A
Female urogenital infections				
Cervix	Cervicitis Or Asymptomatic	Mucopurulent discharge, vaginal pruritus, menorrhagia, bleeding in between menstrual cycles; friable cervical mucosa and frank discharge on physical examination	Pelvic inflammatory disease, chronic pelvic pain, ectopic pregnancy	A normal-appearing cervix does not rule out presence of gonococcal cervicitis
Upper reproductive tract (uterus, ovaries, fallopian tubes)	Pelvic inflammatory disease	Pelvic/abdominal pain, dyspareunia, and abnormal vaginal bleeding; physical examination findings may include abdominal tenderness, uterine tenderness, and adnexal or cervical motion tenderness	Infertility, chronic pelvic pain, ectopic pregnancy	Signs and symptoms are not specific to gonococcal-related PID

All genders				
Rectum	Proctitis Or Asymptomatic	Anorectal bleeding, anorectal pain, tenesmus, constipation, rectal fullness or incomplete defecation, and mucopurulent discharge	Stricture or stenosis, fistulas	N/A
Pharynx	Pharyngitis Or Asymptomatic	Pharyngeal erythema and pain; pharyngeal exudates, cervical lymphadenitis	N/A	N/A
Conjunctiva	Conjunctivitis	Range of severity from conjunctival injection to severe mucopurulent discharge, periorbital edema	Uveitis, severe keratitis; corneal ulceration, perforation, and blindness if left untreated	N/A
Other	Disseminated gonococcal infection	Fevers, chills, malaise, skin lesions (typically described as pustular or vesicopustular, though can be hemorrhagic macules, papules, bullae, and nodules), polyarthralgias, tenosynovitis, arthritis, synovial effusion	Septic arthritis, osteomyelitis; meningitis; endocarditis, can result in significant valvular dysfunction and heart failure	Persons with DGI are often asymptomatic at the mucosal site of infection (urogenital, pharyngeal, and/or rectal site) at the time of clinical presentation

voluntarily reported in the US to CDC between 2020 and 2022, 85.8% required hospitalization, 41.2% underwent related surgeries, and 2.2% died.[31] DGI cases are often asymptomatic at the mucosal site of infection (urogenital, pharyngeal, and/or rectal site) at the time of presentation[32]; thus, clinicians should maintain a high degree of suspicion for patients presenting with signs and symptoms of DGI.

PREVENTION AND CONTROL STRATEGIES

Since the 1970s, gonorrhea prevention and control has relied on screening asymptomatic persons and treating sex partners. Now, 2 novel biomedical prevention strategies are on the horizon—post-exposure prophylaxis (PEP) with doxycycline and a vaccine (See "Novel Approaches and Advances in STI Treatment and Prevention").

Gonorrhea Screening

Given the high proportion of asymptomatic gonorrhea, screening is an important tool for identifying individuals with gonorrhea and providing treatment and other management strategies to reduce the risk of complications and decrease transmission in the community. Recommendations and considerations for gonorrhea screening vary by population, age, and sexual behavior and are published by US Preventive Services Task Force, the CDC, and the HIV Medicine Association of the Infectious Diseases Society of America (See "A Practical Approach to STI Screening for the Primary Care Clinician").

Post-Exposure Prophylaxis with Doxycycline

Randomized controlled trials have evaluated the use of doxycycline taken within 72 hours after sexual activity for the prevention of bacterial sexually transmitted infections (STIs) (ie, chlamydia, gonorrhea, and syphilis), an intervention known as STI PEP.[33] There is concern, however, that early reductions in incident gonorrhea will be followed by major increases in antimicrobial resistance rendering the intervention ineffective for gonorrhea within 10 to 20 years.[34] Additionally, 2 groups have demonstrated that selection for tetracycline resistance also selects for resistance in other antimicrobials which may have more widespread effects on gonorrhea antimicrobial resistance.[35,36]

Vaccination

Gonococcal vaccine research efforts were renewed by the possible protective effects of group B outer membrane vesicle (OMV) meningococcal (MenB) vaccines. In 2017, New Zealand reported a decline in gonorrhea after the large-scale distribution of their meningococcal (MeNZB) vaccine, with an estimated vaccine efficacy of 31%.[37] Other studies using different MenB vaccines have also demonstrated reductions in gonorrhea.[38] Although the MenB vaccine used in New Zealand no longer exists, the 4CMenB, Bexsero (GlaxoSmithKline, UK), vaccine has the same OMV components as the MeNZB vaccine. The impact of meningococcal vaccines on gonococcal infections is promising, but results from additional studies are needed to determine vaccine efficacy and duration of protection.

CLINICAL MANAGEMENT

Gonorrhea Diagnosis

Persons at risk for or suspected of having gonorrhea based on symptoms should undergo evaluation and testing to confirm the microbiologic diagnosis, ensure appropriate treatment, and further management.[39] Diagnostic tests to identify gonorrhea include microscopy, nucleic acid amplification tests (NAAT), and culture; each type has benefits and limitations under different scenarios due to differences in test performance, characteristics, and result turnaround time.

Microscopy

Although not routinely used in current practice, microscopy with Gram stain is a point-of-care (POC) test that can be used with male urethral swabs to differentiate gonococcal urethritis from urethritis due to other pathogens (ie, non-gonococcal urethritis). Gram stain of a male urethral specimen with polymorphonuclear leukocytes with intracellular gram-negative diplococci is highly specific (>95%) and can be considered diagnostic for gonorrhea.[40] Gram stain microscopy is not a reliable tool for diagnosis at any other anatomic sites because of low specificity due to possible presence of other nonpathogenic gram-negative diplococci.[41]

Nucleic Acid Amplification Tests

NAAT are the preferred test for the detection of gonorrhea in patients with or without symptoms given their high sensitivity and specificity and relatively fast turnaround time. NAAT manufacturer product inserts should be reviewed carefully since approved specimen types (eg, urine, urethral, vaginal, cervical) and collection methods, as well as performance, vary by test manufacturer.[39] Two NAAT have been cleared by US Food and Drug Administration (FDA) for detection of gonorrhea and chlamydia from rectal and oropharyngeal samples—Xpert CT/GC Assay (Cepheid, Sunnyvale, CA, USA) and Aptima Combo 2 Assay (Hologic, San Diego, CA, USA), though NAAT from other manufacturers can be used for extragenital specimen collection following laboratory validation. One of the benefits of NAAT is their shelf-stability and ease of use which allow patients to self-collect samples. Patient-collected specimens can be considered for testing outside of clinical spaces.[42]

Point-of-Care Nucleic Acid Amplification Tests

The FDA recently cleared a few near-patient and rapid POC NAAT for the detection of gonorrhea.[43] POC tests allow patients to receive test results and treatment during the same clinic visit. When implemented in places without microscopy or for persons with known sexual exposure to gonorrhea, POC NAAT has the potential to reduce the widespread use of empiric antimicrobials. At present, all gonorrhea POC NAAT are cleared only for urogenital specimens. The GeneXpert assay (Cepheid, Sunnyvale, CA, USA) demonstrated high sensitivity and specificity (95.6%–100% and 99.9%–100%, respectively) for the detection of *N. gonorrhoeae* and *Chlamydia trachomatis* and results in 90 minutes,[44] whereas the Binx io Platform (Binx Health, Limited, Trowbridge, UK and Boston, MA, USA) results in 30 minutes.[45] Both the Gene Xpert and the Binx io require an on-site Clinical Laboratory Improvement Ammendments (CLIA)-certified laboratory and investment in the processing instrument. However, the Visby Medical Sexual Health Test device (Visby Medical, San Jose, CA, USA) is a single-use rapid device approved for detection of *N. gonorrhoeae*, *C. trachomatis*, and *Trichomonas vaginalis* in self-collected vaginal swabs in under 30 minutes.[46] Other POC tests are in development.

Culture

Culture is critical in the management of suspected gonorrhea treatment failures as it is the only testing modality that performs comprehensive antimicrobial susceptibility testing. It is no longer the testing standard in routine clinical care due to lower sensitivity (which varies by anatomic site of infection), long turnaround time, and both clinical and laboratory technical requirements.[47] Although not used routinely, clinics that diagnose gonorrhea should consider a plan for obtaining gonorrhea culture in cases of suspected treatment failure.[39]

Gonorrhea Treatment

Recommended treatment for uncomplicated gonococcal infections

The 2021 CDC STI Treatment Guidelines recommend a single 500 mg intramuscular (IM) dose (for persons weighing $\geq$ 150 kg, a single 1 g IM dose) of ceftriaxone for treatment of uncomplicated urogenital, anorectal, and pharyngeal gonorrhea (**Box 1**).[39] During 2015 to 2020, CDC recommended dual therapy with a single 250 mg IM dose of ceftriaxone and a single 1 g oral dose of azithromycin as first-line treatment of uncomplicated gonococcal infections. The recommendations were re-evaluated and updated in 2020 due to increasing concerns for antimicrobial stewardship and the potential impact of dual therapy on commensal organisms and concurrent STI pathogens, in addition to continued low incidence of ceftriaxone resistance and increased incidence of azithromycin resistance.[7] The rationale for increasing the dose of ceftriaxone to 500 mg was based on recent pharmacokinetics and pharmacodynamics studies of ceftriaxone for gonorrhea treatment.[7] If co-infection with chlamydia has not been excluded, doxycycline 100 mg orally twice daily for 7 days is recommended (or azithromycin 1 g if doxycycline is contraindicated or there are adherence concerns).[39] Persons treated for gonorrhea should abstain from sexual activity for 7 days after treatment and until all sex partners are treated (7 days after receiving treatment and resolution of symptoms if present) to minimize risk of re-infection.[39] All persons diagnosed with gonorrhea should be retested in 3 months due to high rates of reinfection.[39]

Alternative regimens for uncomplicated gonococcal infections

There are currently few reliable alternative antimicrobial treatment regimens for gonorrhea. In cases in which patients report a beta-lactam allergy, it is critical that clinicians first attempt to determine whether it is a true allergy by performing a

Box 1
Recommended and alternative treatment regimens for uncomplicated gonococcal infections

Recommended regimens for uncomplicated gonococcal infections (cervix, urethra, pharynx, or rectum)

Ceftriaxone 500 mg IM as a single dose (*persons weighing <150 kg*)
Ceftriaxone 1 g IM as a single dose (*persons weighing ≥150 kg*)
Test-of-cure is recommended for anyone diagnosed with pharyngeal gonorrhea after initial gonorrhea treatment by using either gonorrhea culture or NAAT

Alternative regimens for uncomplicated gonococcal infection (cervix, urethra, or rectum only)

Gentamicin 240 mg IM as a single dose *plus* azithromycin 2 g orally as a single dose
OR
Cefixime 800 mg orally as a single dose
No reliable alternative treatments are available for pharyngeal gonorrhea
For persons with an anaphylactic or other severe reaction (eg, Stevens-Johnson syndrome) to ceftriaxone, consult an infectious disease specialist

If chlamydial infection has not been excluded

Doxycycline 100 mg orally twice daily for 7 days
OR
Azithromycin 1 g as a single dose (if doxycycline is contraindicated)

thorough patient history (eg, type of reaction, timing of reaction, and previous prescription records) and allergy skin testing.[39] Though the prevalence of reported penicillin allergy has been estimated to be 10% among US population, less than 1% likely have a true penicillin allergy. Clinicians often avoid cephalosporin use (eg, ceftriaxone) in patients with reported penicillin allergies, though the cross-reactivity between penicillin and third-generation cephalosporins is rare.[48,49] Additionally, a majority (80%) of patients with a true IgE-mediated penicillin allergy will lose their hypersensitivity after 10 years[49]; thus, patients with remote allergic reactions may no longer have a hypersensitivity reaction. The use of third-generation cephalosporins (ceftriaxone, cefixime) for the treatment of gonorrhea is safe for patients without a history of any IgE-mediated symptoms (eg, anaphylaxis, urticaria) from penicillin during the preceding 10 years.[39]

For patients with a true beta-lactam allergy and anogenital gonorrhea, the recommended alternative treatment is dual therapy with a single IM gentamicin 240 mg dose and oral azithromycin 2 g once. Though not yet FDA-cleared, laboratory-developed NAAT with gyrase A (gyrA) testing have been shown to be highly sensitive and specific for predicting *N. gonorrhoeae* ciprofloxacin susceptibility.[50] If gyrA testing is available and indicates ciprofloxacin susceptibility, patients with a true beta-lactam allergy can be treated with ciprofloxacin 500 mg orally once.[39] If there are not concerns for a beta-lactam allergy, but ceftriaxone cannot be administered, an 800 mg oral dose of cefixime can be considered as an alternative cephalosporin regimen. Oral cefixime use for the treatment of gonorrhea should be limited as it does not provide the high, sustained bactericidal blood levels as a 500 mg IM dose of ceftriaxone.[39]

There is no recommended alternative regimen for the treatment of pharyngeal gonorrhea. Presently, ceftriaxone is the only available antimicrobial that reliably eradicates gonorrhea at the pharynx.

Future treatments

Historically, public health has relied on new antimicrobial development to overcome gonorrhea's expanding antimicrobial resistance. Zoliflodacin and gepotidacin (new type II topoisomerase inhibitors) have demonstrated *in vitro* activity against *N. gonorrhoeae* with known ciprofloxacin resistance.[51,52] Both drugs are in clinical trials and are expected to be oral therapeutic options for gonorrhea treatment in the relatively near future.

Repurposing currently available drugs is a faster method to new treatments. Ertapenem, a beta-lactam and carbapenem, with demonstrated *in vitro* activity against *N. gonorrhoeae,* was found to be non-inferior to ceftriaxone at anogenital sites in a large randomized controlled trial; however, efficacy against ceftriaxone-resistant strains is uncertain.[53]

Additional Patient Management

Pharyngeal gonorrhea test- of cure

Pharyngeal gonococcal infections consistently have lower cure rates than anogenital gonococcal infections, regardless of antibiotic class. Although this is likely due to variable drug concentrations at the pharynx, including for ceftriaxone, there are many unanswered questions about gonorrhea at this anatomic site. Clinically, most ceftriaxone treatment failures have occurred at the pharynx. Although treatment failure at the pharynx has occurred with susceptible organisms, there have also been treatment failures with strains demonstrating high ceftriaxone MICs (>0.25 μg/mL).[54,55] Due to concerns of potential persistent asymptomatic infection, the unclear penetration of recommended drugs, and the risk of antimicrobial resistance development at the pharynx, the 2021 CDC STI Treatment Guidelines recommended test of cure (TOC) for anyone diagnosed with pharyngeal gonorrhea 7 to 14 days after initial gonorrhea treatment by using either gonorrhea culture or NAAT.[7,39] However, a subsequent study assessing time to clearance of *N. gonorrhoeae* at the pharynx found that positive pharyngeal gonorrhea TOC prior to 12 days after treatment are likely false-positive results, and in the absence of re-exposure, may warrant repeat testing.[56] Prior to retreatment, a confirmatory culture should be attempted for any positive TOC NAAT.[7] All positive TOC cultures should undergo antimicrobial susceptibility testing to assess for resistance.[39] If pharyngeal TOC is persistently NAAT positive and culture negative, clinicians may consider testing on a different NAAT platform since false positives can occur due to cross-reactivity with commensal *Neisseria* species.[47,57]

Management of Sex Partners

Partner notification

Clinicians serve an important role in reducing patients' risk for reinfection by ensuring patients' sex partners are notified of exposure and clinically evaluated.[58] All sex partners from the prior 60 days should be referred for clinical evaluation, testing, and empiric gonorrhea treatment.[39] If the patient's most recent sexual exposure was greater than 60 days before onset of symptoms or diagnosis, the most recent sex partner should be tested and treated for gonorrhea.[39] When feasible, providers should encourage patients to bring their primary sex partner to clinic when returning for treatment so both can be treated concurrently. Providing written information to patients to share with their sex partners can increase rates of partner treatment.[39,59]

Expedited partner therapy

Expedited partner therapy (EPT) is the clinical practice of treating sex partners of persons diagnosed with chlamydia or gonorrhea who are unable or unlikely to seek timely treatment by providing medications to the partner in the absence of a clinical evaluation. EPT is permissible or potentially allowable in all 50 states,[60] and should be offered if the sex partner's access to clinical evaluation and treatment is limited; clinicians should be aware of local EPT regulations.[39] The recommended regimen for gonorrhea EPT is cefixime 800 mg as a single oral dose which can be provided to the partner by the patient or a collaborating pharmacy as permitted by law.[39] The partner should also receive doxycycline 100 mg twice daily for 7 days (or azithromycin 1 g if doxycycline is contraindicated) if the patient has chlamydia or chlamydia has not been ruled out.[39] If the partner is of child-bearing potential and pregnancy status is unknown, azithromycin 1 g for chlamydia EPT can be provided.[61] EPT is supported by evidence from 3 US clinical trials that included heterosexual men and women with gonorrhea or chlamydia and found that more partners were treated when patients were offered EPT and gonorrhea reinfection rates declined.[62,63] There are limited data regarding use of EPT for gonorrhea among MSM. Providers and patients who are MSM should use shared clinical decision-making regarding EPT.[39]

Managing Persistent Gonococcal Infections and Suspected Treatment Failures

Ceftriaxone remains the sole recommended regimen for empiric single-dose gonorrhea treatment but increasing international reports of patients failing ceftriaxone-based therapies have highlighted the need to quickly identify and appropriately treat all suspected treatment failures.[7] The first published report of a gonorrhea ceftriaxone treatment failure occurred in Sweden in 2010.[64] By 2018, the UK reported the first case of a gonococcal treatment failure in the setting of ceftriaxone resistance combined with high-level azithromycin resistance, followed by a similar case in Australia.[7] Although there have been no "resistance-related" ceftriaxone treatment failures identified in the US, gonococcal isolates with high ceftriaxone MIC levels have been reported and public health authorities are concerned about the inevitability of a treatment failure in the US.[65,66]

Suspected gonorrhea treatment failures present either with persistent clinical symptoms or a positive TOC after recommended treatment and in the absence of reinfection (**Table 2**). Alternatively, identification of a concerning laboratory result (ie, antimicrobial MIC value or molecular test result) can lead to suspicions of resistance. Symptomatic persistent infections may lack expected symptom resolution 3 to 5 days after treatment. Asymptomatic persistent infections can only be identified through repeat testing (ie, TOC). Concerning TOC results are either positive cultures greater than 72 hours or positive NAAT greater than 12 (pharyngeal)[56] or NAAT greater than 7 (anogenital) days after recommended treatment.[67]

In the US, reinfections are more likely to occur than true treatment failures. Providers should take a thorough sexual history including asking about timing of symptom resolution, new onset of symptoms, treatment completion and tolerance, abstinence after treatment, treatment of sex partners, and new sex partners since treatment.[68] Additionally, providers should ask regarding recent travel and sexual contacts outside of the US, as most of the internationally reported treatment failures have been associated with travel to Asia.[7,39,64,69] In addition to repeating a gonorrhea NAAT and attempting to perform culture, other sexually transmitted pathogens that produce similar symptoms should be ruled out.[39] Specifically, persistent urogenital symptoms may be due to concurrent infection with *Mycoplasma genitalium* or *T. vaginalis*. Management and treatment next steps should be tailored to the suspected diagnosis.

Once treatment failure is suspected, reinfection is ruled out, and testing has been completed (ie, repeat NAAT and culture specimens obtained), single doses of IM gentamicin 240 mg plus oral azithromycin 2 g can be administered if there is concern that the *N. gonorrhoeae* isolate has an elevated ceftriaxone MIC,[39] though gentamicin is unlikely to be curative for pharyngeal infections.[70] All providers managing a suspected cephalosporin treatment failure are strongly encouraged to consult an infectious disease specialist or an STI clinical expert (https://www.stdccn.org/render/Public) for assistance with clinical management.

Local and state health departments can often help providers with managing suspected gonorrhea treatment failures. Providers are encouraged to communicate with their health departments and public health laboratories. Although culture for *N. gonorrhoeae* should be collected for antimicrobial susceptibility testing,[39] not all laboratories have the capacity to culture *N. gonorrhoeae* or perform susceptibility testing. If local laboratories do not have the capacity to perform this testing, CDC can assist in connecting providers to a laboratory that does. All positive samples should be saved for shipment to CDC through local and state public health mechanisms.[39]

To ensure that potentially resistant strains of gonorrhea are contained, it is important to encourage sex partners to present for testing and treatment, and counsel patients to abstain from sexual activity until their infection has been confirmed to be eradicated. Health departments can help with partner notification and culture evaluation of patients and sex partners with suspected gonorrhea treatment failure.

Table 2
Important considerations when managing a suspected gonococcal treatment failure

Step 1: Evaluate for Persistent Infection		
Symptomatic	*Asymptomatic*	
Patient with persistent symptoms • Symptoms do not resolve (3–5 d) after treatment	Patient with positive test-of-cure (TOC) result(s) • Positive culture (>72 h) after treatment • Positive NAAT (pharyngeal: >12 d or anogenital: >7 d) after treatment	
Step 2: Evaluate for Treatment Failure		
1. Take a thorough sexual history 2. Evaluate for re-exposure to gonorrhea 3. Evaluate for appropriate gonococcal treatment 4. Evaluate for other diagnoses that can present similarly		
Alternative Diagnosis	*Gonococcal Re-infection*	*Suspected Gonococcal Treatment Failure*
Patient with positive test result(s) for another diagnosis • Treat based on diagnosis identified	Patient with positive gonorrhea test result(s), including TOC, when *re-exposure is likely* • Re-treat with initial therapy • If a pharyngeal infection is identified, perform TOC	Patient with positive gonorrhea test result(s), including TOC, when *re-exposure is unlikely* • Prepare for antimicrobial resistance evaluation from all positive anatomic sites • Abnormal laboratory results (ie, antimicrobial MIC value or molecular test result) are managed as suspected treatment failures
Step 3: Evaluate for Antimicrobial Resistance		
1. Contact local/state health department to notify of suspected treatment failure 2. Collect sample for culture and NAAT (simultaneously, unless culture sample(s) already collected as part of TOC) 3. Contact laboratory prior to submission of culture sample for instructions, recommendations, and additional support • If laboratory is unable to perform culture or susceptibility, contact local/state health department for alternative laboratory options • If alternative laboratory options are unknown, contact CDC (gcfailure@cdc.gov) for additional recommendations 4. Submit sample to a laboratory for possible culture growth and resistance testing • Request susceptibility testing be performed (at minimum request testing for ceftriaxone, cefixime, and ciprofloxacin) 5. Consult an infectious disease specialist or an STD clinical expert (https://www.stdccn.org/render/Public) for assistance with clinical management		
Step 4: Management of Suspected Treatment Failure		
Culture positive or NAAT positive result(s) identified		
1. Contact local/state department to notify of culture and NAAT results 2. Health departments can assist with partner investigation, notification, testing, and treatment 3. Save all positive samples (cultures and NAAT), in case additional testing is needed 4. Notify CDC (gcfailure@cdc.gov) and submit case information using the Suspected Gonorrhea Treatment Failure Consultation Form to receive additional recommendations and guidance		

SUMMARY

Gonorrhea rates continue to rise in the US and different populations disproportionally carry the burden of disease. Complicating the management is *N. gonorrhoeae's* propensity to develop resistance to all therapies that have been used for gonococcal treatment. As antimicrobial resistance increases in the US, there are few new antimicrobials being developed. Ceftriaxone is the last remaining highly effective single-dose recommended regimen for gonococcal treatment. The 2021 CDC STI Treatment Guidelines increased the dose of ceftriaxone to 500 mg (1 g if $\geq$ 150 kg) for uncomplicated infections. An increasing number of ceftriaxone-based treatment failures have been reported internationally, most commonly at the pharynx. Therefore, all pharyngeal gonococcal infections are recommended to undergo TOC 7 to 14 days after treatment. It is recommended that all providers, laboratorians, and public health staff become aware of antimicrobial resistant gonorrhea and be able to identify, appropriately manage, and report any suspected gonorrhea treatment failure case.

CLINICS CARE POINTS

- Gonorrhea cases and reported rates continue to increase. National surveillance efforts for gonorrhea and antimicrobial resistant gonorrhea continue to monitor trends across different populations.
- As rates of gonorrhea continue to increase, clinicians will likely see rare clinical presentations of gonorrhea more frequently. Clinicians should maintain a high degree of suspicion for gonorrhea—including rare gonococcal clinical syndromes such as DGI.
- NAAT are considered the preferred test for the detection of gonorrhea in patients with or without symptoms given their high sensitivity and specificity.
- The recommended treatment for uncomplicated gonorrhea in adults and adolescents at urogenital, rectal, and pharyngeal anatomic sites is ceftriaxone 500 mg IM once in a single dose.
- Test of cure is recommended for anyone diagnosed with pharyngeal gonorrhea.
- A reported beta-lactam allergy should prompt a review to determine whether a true allergy is present since there are limited reliable alternative gonorrhea treatment regimens; a very small proportion of the population likely have true penicillin allergies, and the cross-reactivity between penicillin and third-generation cephalosporins is rare.
- If a gonococcal treatment failure is suspected, all efforts should be made to (1) rule out reinfection; (2) obtain simultaneous culture and NAAT samples to evaluate for resistance; (3) provide appropriate treatment after all samples have been collected; and (4) notify state and local health departments. Clinicians should work with local partners to understand policies and procedures for managing suspected treatment failure cases.

DISCLAIMER

The findings and conclusions in this report are those of the authors and do not necessarily represent the official position of the Centers for Disease Control and Prevention (CDC).

DISCLOSURE

S.B. St. Cyr has no conflicts of interest to report. L.A.S. Quilter has no conflicts of interest to report. L.A. Barbee has received research support from Hologic, United States, Nabriva, Ireland and SpeeDx.

REFERENCES

1. Centers for Disease Control and Prevention (CDC). Sexually Transmitted Disease Surveillance Report, 2021. 2022. Available at: https://www.cdc.gov/std/statistics/2021/default.htm. Accessed June 7, 2023.
2. Kreisel KM, Weston EJ, St Cyr SB, et al. Estimates of the Prevalence and Incidence of Chlamydia and Gonorrhea Among US Men and Women, 2018. Sex Transm Dis 2021;48(4):222–31.
3. World Health Organization (WHO). Global health sector strategies on, respectively, HIV, viral hepatitis and sexually transmitted infections for the period 2022-2030. World Health Organization. Available at: https://www.who.int/publications/i/item/9789240053779. Accessed June 7, 2023.
4. Hogben M, Leichliter JS. Social determinants and sexually transmitted disease disparities. Sex Transm Dis 2008;35(12 Suppl):S13–8.
5. Unemo M, Shafer WM. Antibiotic resistance in Neisseria gonorrhoeae: origin, evolution, and lessons learned for the future. Ann N Y Acad Sci 2011;1230:E19–28.
6. Update to CDC's Sexually transmitted diseases treatment guidelines, 2010: oral cephalosporins no longer a recommended treatment for gonococcal infections. MMWR Morb Mortal Wkly Rep 2012;61(31):590–4.
7. Barbee LA, St Cyr SB. Management of Neisseria gonorrhoeae in the United States: Summary of Evidence From the Development of the 2020 Gonorrhea Treatment Recommendations and the 2021 Centers for Disease Control and Prevention Sexually Transmitted Infection Treatment Guidelines. Clin Infect Dis 2022;74(Suppl_2):S95–111.
8. McCormack WM, Stumacher RJ, Johnson K, et al. Clinical spectrum of gonococcal infection in women. Lancet 1977;1(8023):1182–5.
9. Martín-Sánchez M, Ong JJ, Fairley CK, et al. Clinical presentation of asymptomatic and symptomatic heterosexual men who tested positive for urethral gonorrhoea at a sexual health clinic in Melbourne, Australia. BMC Infect Dis 2020;20(1):486.
10. Ong JJ, Fethers K, Howden BP, et al. Asymptomatic and symptomatic urethral gonorrhoea in men who have sex with men attending a sexual health service. Clin Microbiol Infect 2017;23(8):555–9.
11. Handsfield HH, Lipman TO, Harnisch JP, et al. Asymptomatic gonorrhea in men. Diagnosis, natural course, prevalence and significance. N Engl J Med 1974;290(3):117–23.
12. Klouman E, Masenga EJ, Sam NE, et al. Asymptomatic gonorrhoea and chlamydial infection in a population-based and work-site based sample of men in Kilimanjaro, Tanzania. Int J STD AIDS 2000;11(10):666–74.
13. Pelouze PS. Gonorrhea in the Male. Bull N Y Acad Med 1941;17(1):39–44.
14. Eschenbach DA, Buchanan TM, Pollock HM, et al. Polymicrobial etiology of acute pelvic inflammatory disease. N Engl J Med 1975;293(4):166–71.
15. Holmes KK, Eschenbach DA, Knapp JS. Salpingitis: overview of etiology and epidemiology. Am J Obstet Gynecol 1980;138(7 Pt 2):893–900.
16. Chan PA, Robinette A, Montgomery M, et al. Extragenital Infections Caused by Chlamydia trachomatis and Neisseria gonorrhoeae: A Review of the Literature. Infect Dis Obstet Gynecol 2016;2016:5758387.
17. Khosropour CM, Coomes DM, LeClair A, et al. High Prevalence of Rectal Chlamydia and Gonorrhea Among Men Who Have Sex With Men Who Do Not Engage in Receptive Anal Sex. Sex Transm Dis 2023;50(7):404–9.

18. de Vries HJC, Nori AV, Kiellberg Larsen H, et al. European Guideline on the management of proctitis, proctocolitis and enteritis caused by sexually transmissible pathogens. J Eur Acad Dermatol Venereol 2021;35(7):1434–43.
19. Wiesner PJ, Tronca E, Bonin P, et al. Clinical spectrum of pharyngeal gonococcal infection. N Engl J Med 1973;288(4):181–5.
20. Chow EPF, Chen MY, Williamson DA, et al. Oropharyngeal and Genital Gonorrhea Infections Among Women and Heterosexual Men Reporting Sexual Contact With Partners With Gonorrhea: Implication for Oropharyngeal Testing of Heterosexual Gonorrhea Contacts. Sex Transm Dis 2019;46(11):743–7.
21. McLaughlin SE, Golden MR, Soge OO, et al. Pharyngeal Gonorrhea in Heterosexual Male and Female Sex Partners of Persons With Gonorrhea. Sex Transm Dis 2023;50(4):203–8.
22. Charleson F, Tran J, Kolobaric A, et al. A Systematic Review of Kissing as a Risk Factor for Oropharyngeal Gonorrhea or Chlamydia. Sex Transm Dis 2023;50(7): 395–401.
23. Alfonso E, Friedland B, Hupp S, et al. Neisseria gonorrhoeae conjunctivitis. An outbreak during an epidemic of acute hemorrhagic conjunctivitis. JAMA 1983; 250(6):794–5.
24. Mak DB, Smith DW, Harnett GB, et al. A large outbreak of conjunctivitis caused by a single genotype of Neisseria gonorrhoeae distinct from those causing genital tract infections. Epidemiol Infect 2001;126(3):373–8.
25. Laga M, Meheus A, Piot P. Epidemiology and control of gonococcal ophthalmia neonatorum. Bull World Health Organ 1989;67(5):471–7.
26. Hook EW III, Handsfield HH. Gonococcal infections in the adult [Chapter 35]. In: Holmes KK, Sparling PF, Stamm WE, et al, editors. Sexually transmitted diseases. 4th. New York, NY: McGraw-6 Hill Medical; 2008. p. 627–45.
27. Tang EC, Johnson KA, Alvarado L, et al. Characterizing the Rise of Disseminated Gonococcal Infections in California, July 2020-July 2021. Clin Infect Dis 2023; 76(2):194–200.
28. Nettleton WD, Kent JB, Macomber K, et al. Notes from the Field: Ongoing Cluster of Highly Related Disseminated Gonococcal Infections - Southwest Michigan, 2019. MMWR Morb Mortal Wkly Rep 2020;69(12):353–4.
29. Sawatzky P, Martin I, Thorington R, et al. Disseminated Gonococcal Infections in Manitoba, Canada: 2013 to 2020. Sex Transm Dis 2022;49(12):831–7.
30. Merrick R, Pitt R, Enayat Q, et al. National surveillance of disseminated gonococcal infection: preliminary findings from cross-sectional survey data in England, 2016–21. The Lancet. 2021;398:S65. doi:10.1016/S0140-6736(21) 02608-8.
31. Quilter LAS, Tang EC, Johnson KA, et al. Reported disseminated gonococcal infections in the United States, 2020-2022. Presented at: IDWeek 2022; October 21, 2022; Washington, DC.
32. O'Brien JP, Goldenberg DL, Rice PA. Disseminated gonococcal infection: a prospective analysis of 49 patients and a review of pathophysiology and immune mechanisms. Medicine (Baltimore) 1983;62(6):395–406.
33. Luetkemeyer AF, Donnell D, Dombrowski JC, et al. Postexposure Doxycycline to Prevent Bacterial Sexually Transmitted Infections. N Engl J Med 2023;388(14): 1296–306.
34. Reichert E, Grad YH. Resistance and prevalence Implications of doxycycline post-exposure prophylaxis for gonorrhea prevention in men who have sex with men: a modeling study. medRxiv [Preprint] 2023. https://doi.org/10.1101/2023.04.24.23289033.

35. Mortimer TD, Grad YH. A genomic perspective on the near-term impact of doxycycline post-exposure prophylaxis on Neisseria gonorrhoeae antimicrobial resistance. Clin Infect Dis 2023. https://doi.org/10.1093/cid/ciad279.
36. Vanbaelen T, Manoharan-Basil SS, Kenyon C. Doxycycline Post Exposure Prophylaxis could induce cross-resistance to other classes of antimicrobials in Neisseria gonorrhoeae: an in-silico analysis. Sex Transm Dis 2023. https://doi.org/10.1097/olq.0000000000001810.
37. Petousis-Harris H, Paynter J, Morgan J, et al. Effectiveness of a group B outer membrane vesicle meningococcal vaccine against gonorrhoea in New Zealand: a retrospective case-control study. Lancet 2017;390(10102):1603–10.
38. Abara WE, Jerse AE, Hariri S, et al. Planning for a Gonococcal Vaccine: A Narrative Review of Vaccine Development and Public Health Implications. Sex Transm Dis 2021;48(7):453–7.
39. Workowski KA, Bachmann LH, Chan PA, et al. Sexually Transmitted Infections Treatment Guidelines, 2021. MMWR Recomm Rep (Morb Mortal Wkly Rep) 2021;70(4):1–187.
40. Sherrard J, Barlow D. Gonorrhoea in men: clinical and diagnostic aspects. Genitourin Med 1996;72(6):422–6.
41. Goh BT, Varia KB, Ayliffe PF, et al. Diagnosis of gonorrhea by gram-stained smears and cultures in men and women: role of the urethral smear. Sex Transm Dis Jul-Sep 1985;12(3):135–9.
42. Lunny C, Taylor D, Hoang L, et al. Self-Collected versus Clinician-Collected Sampling for Chlamydia and Gonorrhea Screening: A Systemic Review and Meta-Analysis. PLoS One 2015;10(7):e0132776.
43. Gaydos CA, Melendez JH. Point-by-point progress: gonorrhea point of care tests. Expert Rev Mol Diagn 2020;20(8):803–13.
44. Jacobsson S, Boiko I, Golparian D, et al. WHO laboratory validation of Xpert(®) CT/NG and Xpert(®) TV on the GeneXpert system verifies high performances. Apmis 2018;126(12):907–12.
45. Van Der Pol B, Taylor SN, Mena L, et al. Evaluation of the Performance of a Point-of-Care Test for Chlamydia and Gonorrhea. JAMA Netw Open 2020;3(5):e204819.
46. Morris SR, Bristow CC, Wierzbicki MR, et al. Performance of a single-use, rapid, point-of-care PCR device for the detection of Neisseria gonorrhoeae, Chlamydia trachomatis, and Trichomonas vaginalis: a cross-sectional study. Lancet Infect Dis 2021;21(5):668–76.
47. Recommendations for the laboratory-based detection of Chlamydia trachomatis and Neisseria gonorrhoeae–2014. MMWR Recomm Rep 2014;63(Rr-02):1–19.
48. Blumenthal KG, Peter JG, Trubiano JA, et al. Antibiotic allergy. Lancet 2019;393(10167):183–98.
49. Shenoy ES, Macy E, Rowe T, et al. Evaluation and Management of Penicillin Allergy: A Review. JAMA 2019;321(2):188–99.
50. Allan-Blitz LT, Wang X, Klausner JD. Wild-Type Gyrase A Genotype of Neisseria gonorrhoeae Predicts In Vitro Susceptibility to Ciprofloxacin: A Systematic Review of the Literature and Meta-Analysis. Sex Transm Dis 2017;44(5):261–5.
51. Taylor SN, Marrazzo J, Batteiger BE, et al. Single-Dose Zoliflodacin (ETX0914) for Treatment of Urogenital Gonorrhea. N Engl J Med 2018;379(19):1835–45.
52. Taylor SN, Morris DH, Avery AK, et al. Gepotidacin for the Treatment of Uncomplicated Urogenital Gonorrhea: A Phase 2, Randomized, Dose-Ranging, Single-Oral Dose Evaluation. Clin Infect Dis 2018;67(4):504–12.

53. de Vries HJC, de Laat M, Jongen VW, et al. Efficacy of ertapenem, gentamicin, fosfomycin, and ceftriaxone for the treatment of anogenital gonorrhoea (NABOGO): a randomised, non-inferiority trial. Lancet Infect Dis 2022;22(5):706–17.
54. Fifer H, Natarajan U, Jones L, et al. Failure of Dual Antimicrobial Therapy in Treatment of Gonorrhea. N Engl J Med 2016;374(25):2504–6.
55. Eyre DW, Sanderson ND, Lord E, et al. Gonorrhoea treatment failure caused by a Neisseria gonorrhoeae strain with combined ceftriaxone and high-level azithromycin resistance, England. Euro Surveill 2018;23(27). https://doi.org/10.2807/1560-7917.Es.2018.23.27.1800323.
56. Barbee LA, Soge OO, Khosropour CM, et al. Time to Clearance of Neisseria gonorrhoeae RNA at the Pharynx following Treatment. J Clin Microbiol 2022;60(6): e0039922.
57. Hopkins M, Arcenas R, Couto-Parada X, et al. PivNG primers and probes set used in the cobas omni Utility Channel is a reliable supplemental test for detection of Neisseria gonorrhoeae in oropharyngeal, urogenital and rectal specimens collected in cobas PCR Media. Sex Transm Infect 2023. https://doi.org/10.1136/sextrans-2022-055576.
58. Wilson TE, Hogben M, Malka ES, et al. A randomized controlled trial for reducing risks for sexually transmitted infections through enhanced patient-based partner notification. Am J Public Health 2009;99(Suppl 1):S104–10.
59. Trelle S, Shang A, Nartey L, et al. Improved effectiveness of partner notification for patients with sexually transmitted infections: systematic review. BMJ 2007; 334(7589):354.
60. Centers for Disease Control and Prevention (CDC). Legal Status of Expedited Partner Therapy (EPT). 2023. Available at: https://www.cdc.gov/std/ept/legal/default.htm. Accessed June 7, 2023.
61. Public Health - Seattle & King County. Expedited Partner Therapy (EPT) Guidelines. 2022. Available at: https://kingcounty.gov/depts/health/communicable-diseases/hiv-std/providers/partner-notification/ept-guidelines.aspx. Accessed June 7, 2023.
62. Golden MR, Whittington WL, Handsfield HH, et al. Effect of expedited treatment of sex partners on recurrent or persistent gonorrhea or chlamydial infection. N Engl J Med 2005;352(7):676–85.
63. Kissinger PJ, Reilly K, Taylor SN, et al. Early repeat Chlamydia trachomatis and Neisseria gonorrhoeae infections among heterosexual men. Sex Transm Dis 2009;36(8):498–500.
64. Unemo M, Golparian D, Hestner A. Ceftriaxone treatment failure of pharyngeal gonorrhoea verified by international recommendations, Sweden, 2010. Euro Surveill 2011;16(6).
65. Picker MA, Knoblock RJ, Hansen H, et al. Notes from the Field: First Case in the United States of Neisseria gonorrhoeae Harboring Emerging Mosaic penA60 Allele, Conferring Reduced Susceptibility to Cefixime and Ceftriaxone. MMWR Morb Mortal Wkly Rep 2020;69(49):1876–7.
66. Commonwealth of Massachusetts. Press Release: Department of Public Health announces first cases of concerning gonorrhea strain. 2023. Available at: https://www.mass.gov/news/department-of-public-health-announces-first-cases-of-concerning-gonorrhea-strain. Accessed June 7, 2023.
67. Wind CM, Schim van der Loeff MF, Unemo M, et al. Test of Cure for Anogenital Gonorrhoea Using Modern RNA-Based and DNA-Based Nucleic Acid Amplification Tests: A Prospective Cohort Study. Clin Infect Dis 2016;62(11):1348–55.

68. Centers for Disease Control and Prevention (CDC). A Guide to Taking a Sexual History. 2022. Available at: https://www.cdc.gov/std/treatment/sexualhistory.htm. Accessed June 7, 2023.
69. Whiley DM, Jennison A, Pearson J, et al. Genetic characterisation of Neisseria gonorrhoeae resistant to both ceftriaxone and azithromycin. Lancet Infect Dis 2018;18(7):717–8.
70. Barbee LA, Soge OO, Morgan J, et al. Gentamicin Alone Is Inadequate to Eradicate Neisseria Gonorrhoeae From the Pharynx. Clin Infect Dis 2020;71(8): 1877–82.

Mycoplasma genitalium

Key Information for the Primary Care Clinician

Oluyomi A. Obafemi, MD, MPH[a,b], Sarah E. Rowan, MD[a,c], Masayo Nishiyama, RN, DNP[a], Karen A. Wendel, MD[a,c,*]

KEYWORDS

- *Mycoplasma genitalium* • Cervicitis • Urethritis • Nucleic acid amplification test
- Macrolide • Fluoroquinolone • Antimicrobial resistance

KEY POINTS

- *Mycoplasma genitalium* (MG) is an emerging sexually transmitted infection, which appears to be a cause of cervicitis and male urethritis. It may also play a role in pelvic inflammatory disease (PID), epididymitis, proctitis, infertility, adverse outcomes in pregnancy, and human immunodeficiency virus (HIV) transmission.
- Three United States Food and Drug Administration approved nucleic acid amplification tests are available. Testing should be focused and intentional to avoid unnecessary antibiotic use.
- International guidelines for MG testing vary, the Centers for Disease Control and Prevention (CDC) recommends testing for persistent male urethritis, cervicitis, and proctitis. Testing should be considered in cases of PID. Testing is also recommended for sexual contacts of patients with MG. Routine screening in asymptomatic individuals, including pregnant patients, is not recommended.
- There is increasing resistance to macrolides and fluoroquinolones. The use of macrolide resistance assays can help guide therapy, but resistance tests are not widely available in the United States.
- The CDC recommends 2-step treatment with doxycycline followed by either azithromycin if resistance testing is available and demonstrates sensitivity to macrolides or moxifloxacin if resistance testing is unavailable or macrolide resistance is detected.

INTRODUCTION

Although *Mycoplasma genitalium* (MG) was first described in 1981 in association with male urethritis, the natural history and the significance of this sexually transmitted infection (STI) remains incompletely understood.[1,2] Over the last four decades, data have linked MG with acute genital tract disease, proctitis, infertility, pregnancy complications, and human immunodeficiency virus (HIV) infection. Expanding access to

[a] Public Health Institute at Denver Health, 601 Broadway, 8th Floor, MC 2800, Denver, CO 80203-3407, USA; [b] Department of Family Medicine, University of Colorado Denver, Aurora, CO, USA; [c] Division of Infectious Diseases, Department of Medicine, University of Colorado Denver, Aurora, CO, USA

* Corresponding author. Public Health Institute at Denver Health, 601 Broadway, 8th floor, MC 2800, Denver, CO 80203-3407.

E-mail address: karen.wendel@dhha.org

Med Clin N Am 108 (2024) 297–310
https://doi.org/10.1016/j.mcna.2023.07.004
medical.theclinics.com

diagnostic testing and growing concerns about antimicrobial resistance (AR) have fueled debate on when to test for MG and how to manage infection. This article will review the current state of knowledge for MG and clinical guidance for care. Given the limited data on MG in transgender people, the terms “men/male” and “women/female” in this article refer to persons assigned male and female at birth.

BACKGROUND

MG is part of a unique group of slow growing, fastidious organisms that lack a cell wall.[1] MG binds to urogenital epithelium, and through surface-exposed lipoproteins, it elicits proinflammatory signals that result in local inflammation and recruitment of monocytes/macrophages and neutrophils.[3] Although infection can resolve without antibiotic therapy, the organism has been demonstrated to persist for months to over a year.[4-6] Persistent infection is likely facilitated by immunologic evasion through its capacity for extensive antigenic variation.[7] Due to limited treatment options and emerging MG AR, the Centers for Disease Control and Prevention (CDC) added drug-resistant MG to its Antibiotic Resistant Threats in the United States, 2019, Watch List.[8]

EPIDEMIOLOGY

The prevalence of MG varies across populations. In a meta-analysis, the estimated prevalence of MG in the general population was 1.3% in highly developed countries and 3.86% in countries with low to medium development indices with no significant difference between men and women.[9] In men who have sex with men (MSM), estimated MG prevalence was higher in the rectum (6.2%) and urethra (5.0%) than the pharynx (1.0%).[10] Co-infection has been described with other bacterial STIs and *Trichomonas vaginalis* (TV).[11,12] In the United States, elevated MG rates are associated with younger age and black race raising concerns about the impact of social determinants of health on MG infection.[12-15]

CLINICAL RELEVANCE

Data linking MG to clinical disease are primarily cross-sectional with limited reports from animal models and longitudinal retrospective studies. As a result, conclusions about causality have been limited. The two clinical conditions most closely linked with MG infection are urethritis in men and cervicitis in women, but limited data also raise concern for associations with upper genital tract disease, proctitis, infertility, pregnancy complications, and HIV acquisition and transmission.

Urethritis

MG has been identified as a cause of both symptomatic and asymptomatic male urethritis.[16-19] Symptoms of MG urethritis are typically mild and often clinically indistinguishable from chlamydial urethritis and other causes of nongonococcal urethritis (NGU). MG has been identified in 15% to 31% of men with symptomatic NGU and has been found in 20% to 25% of cases of non-chlamydial NGU.[17,20–22] After *Chlamydia trachomatis* (CT), MG is the most common cause of NGU.[17,19,21] Urethritis with MG and CT coinfection can also occur.[16,19] Primate models have bolstered the case for causality demonstrating development of urethritis in primates inoculated with MG.[23] Finally, a recent study demonstrated a reduction in clinic visits for persistent NGU after implementing doxycycline as first-line therapy and MG testing at initial presentation of NGU with further treatment for those with a positive MG test.[24] More data are needed, but these results suggest a possible benefit to testing and treating for MG in men presenting with NGU.

Balanitis, Posthitis, Epididymitis, and Prostatitis

There is little data linking MG with other male urogenital syndromes. Although one trial described an association of MG with balanitis and/or posthitis (ie, inflammation of the foreskin), it did not control for candida infection.[25] Similarly, MG has rarely been identified in cases of epididymitis and has not been identified as an independent cause of prostatitis.[26,27]

Cervicitis

MG is identified in 10% to 30% of clinical cases of cervicitis, and data across multiple studies demonstrate an association of MG with acute cervicitis, both independently and as a copathogen with CT or other bacteria.[18,28-32] A study of chronic MG in women with HIV demonstrated increased pro-inflammatory cytokines and inflammatory cervical infiltrates that normalized after MG treatment.[33] Despite some mixed results of animal studies, MG has not been consistently linked to isolated vaginitis or vaginal symptoms.[34,35] Detection of MG in vaginal fluids is generally thought to represent shedding from cervical infection as is seen with CT and *Neisseria gonorrhoeae* (NG).[36]

Pelvic Inflammatory Disease (PID)

MG has been identified in 6% to 33% of women with PID.[37] In a meta-analysis, MG was associated with PID with persistent significant association after accounting for coinfections.[38] However, a meta-analysis of two prospective studies demonstrated a trend toward higher incidence of PID in people with MG but did not reach statistical significance or prove causality.[5] Notably, in a case-control study evaluating postabortal PID, 12.2% of the women with MG prior to medical and surgical termination developed PID as compared to 2.4% who were MG and CT negative ($P = .01$).[39] This strong association has sparked interest in screening and treatment of MG prior to termination of pregnancy.

The importance of MG in the management of PID remains unclear. A retrospective study failed to demonstrate superior microbiological cure (95% for each group) for MG-associated PID treated with moxifloxacin versus standard therapy despite improved clinical cure (89% vs 53% for standard therapy; $P = .004$).[40]

Infertility and Adverse Pregnancy Outcomes

Male infertility has not been linked to MG, but studies in women suggest a possible association and a need for more rigorous investigation. Physiologically, the greatest concern is for MG-mediated tubal factor infertility.[41] Although a meta-analysis of five studies failed to demonstrate a significant association between female infertility and MG infection, after limiting evaluation to three studies that accounted for coinfection, the pooled odds ratio (OR) was 3.27 (95% CI 1.25–8.57).[38] More recently, a meta-analysis that excluded serologic studies suggested a strong association (OR 13.03; 95% CI 3.46–48.98).[42] In a prospective cohort study, serologic evidence of MG infection was associated with infertility as well as a longer median time to conception.[43]

Three meta-analyses have found associations between MG and risk of preterm birth.[38,42,44] Studies linking MG infection with ectopic pregnancy have been inconclusive.[45,46] Spontaneous abortion, premature rupture of membranes, and low birth weight have not been associated with MG infection.[42,44]

There are no data currently available to suggest that screening and treating for MG in asymptomatic women leads to long-term reductions in cervicitis, PID, infertility or poor obstetric outcomes.

Extragenital Mycoplasma genitalium: Rectal Infection, Proctitis, and Pharyngitis

Studies evaluating male proctitis have demonstrated MG-monoinfection in 5.6% to 17% of cases, but studies have not consistently identified an association of rectal MG with symptoms of proctitis.[47-49] A meta-analysis assessing rectal MG infection identified a higher prevalence of MG infection in men with rectal symptoms than in men without.[10] Overall, data on the role of MG in proctitis remain inconclusive and require further study. Oropharyngeal colonization with MG is uncommon and typically not associated with symptoms.[10]

Mycoplasma genitalium and Human Immunodeficiency Virus

People with HIV (PWH) have a higher prevalence of MG, including symptomatic MG infection.[49] A natural history study of banked cervical swabs showed a delayed clearance of untreated MG in women with HIV compared to women without HIV.[50] The role of HIV viremia in delaying clearance has not been evaluated. Thus, it is unclear if higher rates of MG occur among PWH with suppressed viral loads. Female MG urogenital infection has been identified as a risk factor for HIV acquisition.[51,52] In addition, in women with untreated HIV, MG infection has been independently associated with detection of genital HIV RNA.[53]

EVALUATION

Screening

Although screening asymptomatic women for CT can prevent serious sequelae such as PID, no currently available data exist to suggest a benefit from treating asymptomatic MG.[54] In fact, given current challenges posed by MG-AR and limited therapeutic options, there are concerns that asymptomatic MG treatment could result in further evolution of AR and potential barriers to managing symptomatic infection. Therefore, screening for MG is only currently recommended in sexual contacts of people with symptomatic MG (**Table 1**).[55-58] Routine screening of asymptomatic individuals who are not contacts, including pregnant individuals, is not recommended.

Diagnostic Testing

With limited quality of evidence linking MG to various STI syndromes, guidelines for the use of MG diagnostic testing vary. The CDC recommends MG testing for recurrent NGU, cervicitis, and proctitis and testing for sexual contacts of a person with MG infection.[55] MG testing should be considered in patients with PID. US-based providers are advised to follow CDC guidelines. However, recommendations from other countries differ. A summary of current international guidelines for MG testing is provided in **Table 1** for comparison.[55-59]

Test of Cure (TOC)

Current CDC guidelines recommend a TOC if symptoms of infection fail to resolve after treatment or if a patient was treated with doxycycline followed by azithromycin without resistance testing.[55] In addition to testing patients with persistent symptoms, Canadian guidelines recommend a TOC for patients living in regions that have high levels of antimicrobial resistance.[59] European and British guidelines recommend a TOC in all patients, and Australian guidelines recommend TOC for unresolved symptoms or ongoing risk of reinfection or sequelae.[56-58] The optimal timing of TOC is unknown. Limited data suggest that the majority of MG nucleic acid amplification tests (NAATs) may clear within 8 days, but early testing has the potential for false-positive and false-negative results. False-negative results can occur due to transient low

Table 1
Recommendations for testing for *Mycoplasma genitalium:* CDC guidelines for US providers with comparison to international guidelines[55–59]

	U.S.	Canada	UK	Europe	Australia
General screening in asymptomatic patients is not recommended by any guidelines					
Testing of sexual contacts to MG	+	-	+	+	+
Urethritis	-	-	+	+	+
Only recurrent/persistent urethritis	+	+[a]	-	-	+
Epididymitis	-	-	C	+[b]	-
Only recurrent/persistent epididymitis	-	-	-	-	-
Cervicitis	-	-	C	+	+
Only recurrent/persistent cervicitis	+	+[a]	-	-	-
PID	C	-	+	+	+
Only recurrent/persistent PID	-	+[a]	-	-	-
Post coital bleeding	-	-	C	+	+
Dysuria in women	-	-	-	+[c]	-
Proctitis/anal symptoms	-	-	C	+[d]	C
Only recurrent/persistent proctitis	+	-	-	-	-
Prior to termination of pregnancy	-	-	-	C	-

+, recommended; - no recommendation; C, Consider.
[a] When gonorrhea and chlamydia have been ruled out.
[b] Epididymitis in males aged <50 years.
[c] Dysuria with no known other etiology.
[d] Proctitis with negative gonorrhea and chlamydia testing.

organism loads, especially in the setting of evolving AR.[60] Therefore, performing a TOC 3 to 4 weeks after therapy may be preferable.

Mycoplasma genitalium Tests

Microscopy of urethral discharge is not useful in the diagnosis of MG. MG culture is not widely available and can require weeks to months to complete.[55] Serologic tests have not been approved by the Food and Drug Administration (FDA). As a result, NAATs are recommended for the diagnosis of MG.

There are three MG NAATs that are FDA approved for use in clinical settings: Aptima *Mycoplasma genitalium* Assay (Hologic Inc), Cobas TV/MG (Roche Molecular Systems, Inc), which tests for TV and MG, and Alinity m STI Assay (Abbott Molecular, Inc), which tests for CT, NG, MG, and TV.[61] The Aptima and Cobas tests are approved for use with urine, self-collected vaginal or penile meatal swabs, and clinician-collected vaginal, endocervical, or male urethral swabs. The Alinity test is approved for male urine, endocervical swabs, and clinician-collected and self-collected vaginal swabs. Vaginal swabs have the highest sensitivity for MG detection in women followed by endocervical and urine samples.[62] First-catch urine is the preferred sample in men.[63] Some clinical labs in the United States use non-FDA approved lab-developed tests. These tests may have reduced reliability.[63]

In patients with MG-positive NAATs, the CDC and other guideline groups recommend molecular testing for AR.[55-58] Several single nucleotide polymorphisms (SNPs) in the 23S rRNA of MG have been identified as macrolide-resistance–associated mutations (MRMs).[64,65] These MRMs are clearly associated with azithromycin treatment failure. Several Conformité Européene (CE)-marked MRM tests that include multiple SNPs are available in other countries, but none are FDA approved or widely available for commercial use in the United States.[63]

MG fluoroquinolone resistance is conferred by mutations in topoisomerase IV (*parC*) and DNA gyrase (*gyrA*).[63] The most common MG *parC* mutation is associated with a moxifloxacin failure rate of 62.5%.[66] Rates of treatment failure to moxifloxacin may increase to 81% in the setting of dual *parC* and *gyrA* mutations.[67] There are no FDA approved MG fluoroquinolone resistance assays, and commercial tests currently only target *parC* mutations.

Therapeutic Options/Antimicrobial Resistance

Treatment options for MG are limited. Efficacy of doxycycline monotherapy is between 31% and 45%.[68,69] Doxycycline minimum inhibitory concentrations for MG are not associated with clearance of infection, and as a result, factors associated with doxycycline treatment failure are poorly understood.[70] Similarly, the efficacy of azithromycin single-dose therapy has been decreasing with increased prevalence of MRMs.[71-73] Global MRMs increased from 10% before 2010 to 51% in 2016 to 2017.[74] In the United States, MRMs have been identified in 64.4% of the men in STI clinics and 31% to 41% of pregnant women.[12,15,75]

Moxifloxacin is the preferred treatment for macrolide-resistant MG. However, data from Australia demonstrate an increase in *parC* mutations from 13% in 2012 to 2013 to 23% in 2019 to 2020.[76] In the United States, the prevalence of fluoroquinolone resistance mutations has varied from approximately 11% in heterosexual couples and men with urethritis to 40% in rectal samples and 26.7% in urogenital samples from MSM living with HIV.[75,77,78] Of great concern are reports identifying 68.3% prevalence of fluoroquinolone mutations in MSM in Japan and 89.5% prevalence of *parC* mutations in men with urethritis in China.[79,80] Overall, these data align with a meta-analysis of MG treatment demonstrating a decrease in moxifloxacin efficacy from 100% to 89% when comparing studies before and after 2010.[81]

Resistance-Guided and 2-Stage Therapy

Recently, attention has turned to macrolide resistance–guided therapy (RGT) and 2-stage therapy (TST) with doxycycline followed by a macrolide or fluoroquinolone. RGT for MRMs is recommended by multiple guideline groups to determine which patients should be treated with azithromycin or moxifloxacin.[55–58] Initial doxycycline is given in TST in an attempt to lower organism load, improve therapeutic efficacy, and reduce evolution of AR.[82,83] A study combining RGT and TST with doxycycline followed by azithromycin or moxifloxacin demonstrated a microbial cure in 95% of the patients treated with azithromycin and 92% of the patients treated with moxifloxacin.[83]

The CDC recommends testing for MRMs if testing is available. If macrolide resistance testing is negative, patients should be treated with doxycycline 100 mg orally twice daily for 7 days followed by azithromycin 1 g orally initial dose, followed by 500 mg orally once daily for 3 additional days (**Fig. 1**).[55] If macrolide resistance testing is unavailable or demonstrates macrolide-resistant MG, treatment should be doxycycline 100 mg orally twice daily for 7 days followed by moxifloxacin 400 mg orally once daily for 7 days. These recommendations align with Australian STI guidelines.[58] British and European guidelines recommend RGT but differ on recommendations for TST and azithromycin dosing.[56,57]

Options for treatment during pregnancy are limited. Doxycycline may cause tooth discoloration and is therefore contraindicated after the first trimester of pregnancy.[55] Use of moxifloxacin, like other fluoroquinolones, is not recommended in pregnancy due to concerns about cartilage and joint damage in the neonate.[2,55] If MG is known to be macrolide susceptible or if resistance testing is not available, patients with uncomplicated disease can be treated with azithromycin alone with consideration for TOC. For complicated disease or evidence of treatment failure after azithromycin therapy, consider expert consultation as outlined in the following paragaphs.

Partner Testing & Treatment

MG infection occurs in 39% to 50% of heterosexual couples and in 27% of MSM partners.[5] Most guidelines recommend MG testing for current or ongoing partner(s) of a patient with MG.[55–58] Partners with MG or who are unable to access MG testing should be treated with the same antimicrobial regimen as the patient.[55]

Treatment Failure/Persistent Symptoms

If a patient fails moxifloxacin-based therapy and persistent infection is confirmed (see TOC above), alternative therapies are limited, and expert consultation is advised. Minocycline is available in the United States and is recommended at 100 mg twice daily for 14 days. Cure rates are reported to be between 68% and 71%.[2,84] In vitro data suggest lefamulin, omadacycline, and tinidazole have activity against MG, but these medications remain clinically unproven.[85–87] Pristinamycin and sitafloxacin are not available in the United States but have been found to have clinical efficacy.[88,89]

Expert consultation is available for patients with MG treatment failure through the online U.S. National Network of Prevention Training Center's STD Clinical Consultation Network (https://www.stdccn.org). In addition, the CDC maintains a *Mycoplasma genitalium* Treatment Failure Registry (https://airc.cdc.gov/surveys/?s=7NCDWJAYF7ML4PRK)) to collect clinical information on cases of MG that fail antimicrobial therapy.

DISCUSSION & SUMMARY

MG has been detected in 1.3% to 3.86% of the general population but prevalence can be as high as 26% in select groups attending STD clinics.[9,90] Although MG has been

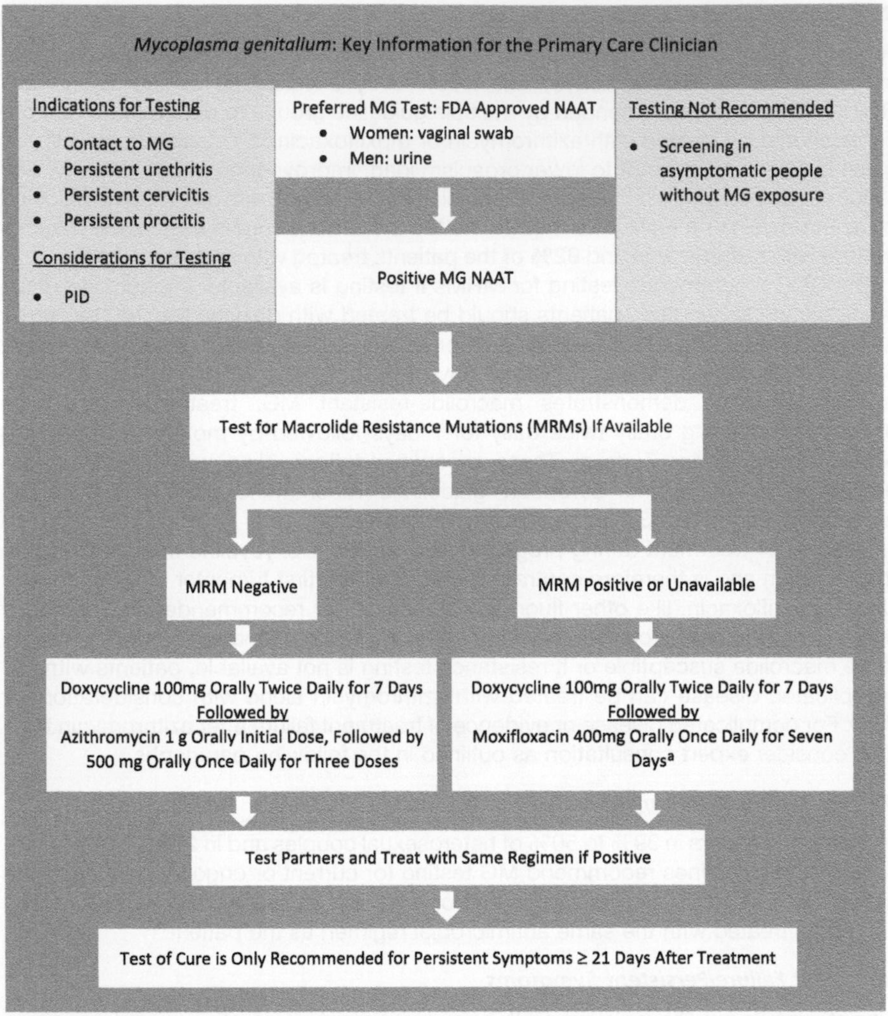

Fig. 1. Diagnosis and management of *Mycoplasma genitalium* (MG). Based on CDC STI treatment guidelines 2021. FDA, Food and Drug Administration; MG, *Mycoplasma genitalium*; MRM, macrolide resistance mutation; NAAT, nucleic acid amplification test; PID, pelvic inflammatory disease. [a]Treatment regimen for uncomplicated disease. If treating PID, treat with moxifloxacin for 14 days. (*From* Workowski KA, Bachmann LH, Chan PA, et al. Sexually Transmitted Infections Treatment Guidelines, 2021. MMWR Recomm Rep. 2021;70(4):1-187. Published 2021 Jul 23. https://doi.org/10.15585/mmwr.rr7004a1.)

associated with several syndromes of urogenital disease, causality is best established for male urethritis and cervicitis. Further research is needed to determine if identifying and treating MG will improve outcomes in PID, epididymitis, proctitis, or pregnancy and if MG diagnosis and treatment will reduce infertility or HIV transmission.

The availability of reliable, FDA approved NAATs for MG diagnosis and the inclusion of specific recommendations for MG testing and treatment in the CDC STI Treatment Guidelines, 2021, will likely increase provider awareness and appropriate MG diagnosis and treatment. However, treatment remains complicated due to increasing resistance, limited therapeutic options, and lack of access to resistance testing.

It is imperative that providers are aware of the importance of focused MG testing to maximize benefits to patients and reduce risks of antibiotic side effects and further evolution of MG-AR.[91] Asymptomatic infection is common. The use of MG tests for asymptomatic screening or in the evaluation of syndromes not clearly linked to MG infection is not of proven benefit to patients and could result in increased AR and antibiotic-associated toxicity. Further research is needed to define the natural history of MG infection and the clinical impact of antimicrobial therapy. Access to improved molecular resistance tests may also lead to optimized approaches to treatment and aid in the control and prevention of MG-associated morbidity. Knowledge about MG and its optimal management is evolving. Clinicians should stay abreast of new recommendations for testing and treatment by reviewing CDC STI treatment guidelines and updates.

CLINICS CARE POINTS

- International guidelines for MG testing vary, the CDC recommends testing for persistent male urethritis, cervicitis, and proctitis. Testing should be considered in cases of PID. Testing is also recommended for sexual contacts of patients with MG.
- Screening asymptomatic people without known MG exposure is not recommended due to the absence of data demonstrating a benefit of treatment and concerns about evolving antimicrobial resistance.
- When possible, providers should use FDA approved MG NAATs and, if available, test for macrolide resistance mutations to guide therapy.
- The CDC recommends 2-step therapy treating with doxycycline followed by azithromycin or moxifloxacin based on resistance testing. If resistance testing is unavailable, the CDC recommends doxycycline followed by moxifloxacin therapy.

DISCLOSURES

K. Wendel receives research funding from Hologic, Inc for evaluation of *M genitalium* prevalence and antimicrobial resistance. There are no other conflicts to report for the authors.

REFERENCES

1. Tully JG, Taylor-Robinson D, Cole RM, et al. A newly discovered mycoplasma in the human urogenital tract. Lancet 1981;1(8233):1288–91.
2. Wood GE, Bradshaw CS, Manhart LE. Update in Epidemiology and Management of Mycoplasma genitalium Infections. Infect Dis Clin North Am 2023;37(2):311–33.
3. McGowin CL, Totten PA. The unique microbiology and molecular pathogenesis of mycoplasma genitalium. J Infect Dis 2017;216(suppl_2):S382–8.
4. Oakeshott P, Aghaizu A, Hay P, et al. Is Mycoplasma genitalium in women the "New Chlamydia?" A community-based prospective cohort study. Clin Infect Dis 2010;51(10):1160–6.
5. Cina M, Baumann L, Egli-Gany D, et al. *Mycoplasma genitalium* incidence, persistence, concordance between partners and progression: systematic review and meta-analysis. Sex Transm Infect 2019;95(5):328–35.
6. Seña AC, Lee JY, Schwebke J, et al. A silent epidemic: the prevalence, incidence and persistence of mycoplasma genitalium among young, asymptomatic high-risk women in the United States. Clin Infect Dis 2018;67(1):73–9.

7. Ma L, Mancuso M, Williams JA, et al. Extensive variation and rapid shift of the MG192 sequence in Mycoplasma genitalium strains from patients with chronic infection. Infect Immun 2014;82(3):1326–34.
8. CDC. Antibiotic resistance Threats in the United States, 2019. Atlanta, GA: U.S. Department of Health and Human Services, CDC; 2019.
9. Baumann L, Cina M, Egli-Gany D, et al. Prevalence of *Mycoplasma genitalium* in different population groups: systematic review and meta-analysis. Sex Transm Infect 2018;94(4):255–62.
10. Latimer RL, Shilling HS, Vodstrcil LA, et al. Prevalence of *Mycoplasma genitalium* by anatomical site in men who have sex with men: a systematic review and meta-analysis. Sex Transm Infect 2020;96(8):563–70.
11. Munson E, Bykowski H, Munson KL, et al. Clinical Laboratory Assessment of Mycoplasma genitalium Transcription-Mediated Amplification Using Primary Female Urogenital Specimens. J Clin Microbiol 2016;54(2):432–8.
12. Stafford IA, Hummel K, Dunn JJ, et al. Retrospective analysis of infection and antimicrobial resistance patterns of *Mycoplasma genitalium* among pregnant women in the southwestern USA. BMJ Open 2021;11(6):e050475.
13. Manhart LE, Gaydos CA, Taylor SN, et al. Characteristics of Mycoplasma genitalium Urogenital Infections in a Diverse Patient Sample from the United States: Results from the Aptima Mycoplasma genitalium Evaluation Study (AMES). J Clin Microbiol 2020;58(7). 001655-20.
14. Gaydos CA, Manhart LE, Taylor SN, et al. Molecular Testing for Mycoplasma genitalium in the United States: Results from the AMES Prospective Multicenter Clinical Study. J Clin Microbiol 2019;57(11). 011255-e1219.
15. Hu M, Souder JP, Subramaniam A, et al. Prevalence of Mycoplasma genitalium infection and macrolide resistance in pregnant women receiving prenatal care. Int J Gynaecol Obstet 2023;160(1):341–4.
16. Mena L, Wang X, Mroczkowski TF, et al. Mycoplasma genitalium infections in asymptomatic men and men with urethritis attending a sexually transmitted diseases clinic in New Orleans. Clin Infect Dis 2002;35(10):1167–73.
17. Falk L, Fredlund H, Jensen JS. Symptomatic urethritis is more prevalent in men infected with Mycoplasma genitalium than with Chlamydia trachomatis. Sex Transm Infect 2004;80(4):289–93.
18. Anagrius C, Loré B, Jensen JS. Mycoplasma genitalium: prevalence, clinical significance, and transmission. Sex Transm Infect 2005;81(6):458–62.
19. Moi H, Reinton N, Moghaddam A. Mycoplasma genitalium is associated with symptomatic and asymptomatic non-gonococcal urethritis in men. Sex Transm Infect 2009;85(1):15–8.
20. Taylor-Robinson D, Jensen JS. Mycoplasma genitalium: from Chrysalis to multicolored butterfly. Clin Microbiol Rev 2011;24(3):498–514.
21. Seña AC, Lensing S, Rompalo A, et al. Chlamydia trachomatis, Mycoplasma genitalium, and Trichomonas vaginalis infections in men with nongonococcal urethritis: predictors and persistence after therapy. J Infect Dis 2012;206(3):357–65.
22. Gaydos C, Maldeis NE, Hardick A, et al. Mycoplasma genitalium compared to chlamydia, gonorrhoea and trichomonas as an aetiological agent of urethritis in men attending STD clinics. Sex Transm Infect 2009;85(6):438–40.
23. Tully JG, Taylor-Robinson D, Rose DL, et al. Urogenital challenge of primate species with Mycoplasma genitalium and characteristics of infection induced in chimpanzees. J Infect Dis 1986;153(6):1046–54.
24. Johnson KA, Sankaran M, Kohn RP, et al. Testing for Mycoplasma genitalium and Using Doxycycline as First-Line Therapy at Initial Presentations for Non-

Gonococcal Urethritis (NGU) Correlate With Reductions in Persistent NGU. Clin Infect Dis 2023;76(9):1674–7.
25. Horner PJ, Taylor-Robinson D. Association of Mycoplasma genitalium with balanoposthitis in men with non-gonococcal urethritis. Sex Transm Infect 2011;87(1):38–40.
26. Eickhoff JH, Frimodt-Møller N, Walter S, et al. A double-blind, randomized, controlled multicentre study to compare the efficacy of ciprofloxacin with pivampicillin as oral therapy for epididymitis in men over 40 years of age. BJU Int 1999;84(7):827–34.
27. Ito S, Tsuchiya T, Yasuda M, et al. Prevalence of genital mycoplasmas and ureaplasmas in men younger than 40 years-of-age with acute epididymitis. Int J Urol 2012;19(3):234–8.
28. Oliphant J, Azariah S. Cervicitis: limited clinical utility for the detection of Mycoplasma genitalium in a cross-sectional study of women attending a New Zealand sexual health clinic. Sex Health 2013;10(3):263–7.
29. Mobley VL, Hobbs MM, Lau K, et al. Mycoplasma genitalium infection in women attending a sexually transmitted infection clinic: diagnostic specimen type, coinfections, and predictors. Sex Transm Dis 2012;39(9):706–9.
30. Gaydos C, Maldeis NE, Hardick A, et al. Mycoplasma genitalium as a contributor to the multiple etiologies of cervicitis in women attending sexually transmitted disease clinics. Sex Transm Dis 2009;36(10):598–606.
31. Manhart LE, Critchlow CW, Holmes KK, et al. Mucopurulent cervicitis and Mycoplasma genitalium. J Infect Dis 2003;187(4):650–7 [published correction appears in J Infect Dis. 2004 Aug 15;190(4):866].
32. Lusk MJ, Konecny P, Naing ZW, et al. Mycoplasma genitalium is associated with cervicitis and HIV infection in an urban Australian STI clinic population. Sex Transm Infect 2011;87(2):107–9.
33. Dehon PM, Hagensee ME, Sutton KJ, et al. Histological Evidence of Chronic Mycoplasma genitalium-Induced Cervicitis in HIV-Infected Women: A Retrospective Cohort Study. J Infect Dis 2016;213(11):1828–35.
34. Latimer RL, Vodstrcil LA, Plummer EL, et al. The clinical indications for testing women for *Mycoplasma genitalium*. Sex Transm Infect 2022;98(4):277–85.
35. Aguila LKT, Patton DL, Gornalusse GG, et al. Ascending reproductive tract infection in pig-tailed macaques inoculated with mycoplasma genitalium. Infect Immun 2022;90(6):e0013122.
36. Wiesenfeld HC, Manhart LE. Mycoplasma genitalium in Women: Current Knowledge and Research Priorities for This Recently Emerged Pathogen. J Infect Dis 2017;216(suppl_2):S389–95.
37. Mitchell CM, Anyalechi GE, Cohen CR, et al. Etiology and Diagnosis of Pelvic Inflammatory Disease: Looking Beyond Gonorrhea and Chlamydia. J Infect Dis 2021;224(12 Suppl 2):S29–35.
38. Lis R, Rowhani-Rahbar A, Manhart LE. Mycoplasma genitalium infection and female reproductive tract disease: a meta-analysis. Clin Infect Dis 2015;61(3):418–26.
39. Bjartling C, Osser S, Persson K. The association between Mycoplasma genitalium and pelvic inflammatory disease after termination of pregnancy. BJOG 2010;117(3):361–4.
40. Latimer RL, Read TRH, Vodstrcil LA, et al. Clinical features and therapeutic response in women meeting criteria for presumptive treatment for pelvic inflammatory disease associated with mycoplasma genitalium. Sex Transm Dis 2019;46(2):73–9.

41. Manhart LE, Broad JM, Golden MR. Mycoplasma genitalium: should we treat and how? Clin Infect Dis 2011;53(Suppl 3):S129–42.
42. Ma C, Du J, Dou Y, et al. The associations of genital mycoplasmas with female infertility and adverse pregnancy outcomes: a systematic review and meta-analysis. Reprod Sci 2021;28(11):3013–31.
43. Peipert JF, Zhao Q, Schreiber CA, et al. Intrauterine device use, sexually transmitted infections, and fertility: a prospective cohort study. Am J Obstet Gynecol 2021;225(2):157.e1–9.
44. Frenzer C, Egli-Gany D, Vallely LM, et al. Adverse pregnancy and perinatal outcomes associated with *Mycoplasma genitalium:* systematic review and meta-analysis. Sex Transm Infect 2022;98(3):222–7.
45. Jurstrand M, Jensen JS, Magnuson A, et al. A serological study of the role of Mycoplasma genitalium in pelvic inflammatory disease and ectopic pregnancy. Sex Transm Infect 2007;83(4):319–23.
46. Ashshi AM, Batwa SA, Kutbi SY, et al. Prevalence of 7 sexually transmitted organisms by multiplex real-time PCR in Fallopian tube specimens collected from Saudi women with and without ectopic pregnancy. BMC Infect Dis 2015;15:569.
47. Read TRH, Murray GL, Danielewski JA, et al. Symptoms, sites, and significance of mycoplasma genitalium in men who have sex with men. Emerg Infect Dis 2019;25(4):719–27.
48. Ong JJ, Aung E, Read TRH, et al. Clinical characteristics of anorectal mycoplasma genitalium infection and microbial cure in men who have sex with men. Sex Transm Dis 2018;45(8):522–6.
49. Soni S, Alexander S, Verlander N, et al. The prevalence of urethral and rectal Mycoplasma genitalium and its associations in men who have sex with men attending a genitourinary medicine clinic. Sex Transm Infect 2010;86(1):21–4.
50. Vandepitte J, Weiss HA, Kyakuwa N, et al. Natural history of *Mycoplasma genitalium* infection in a cohort of female sex workers in Kampala, Uganda. Sex Transm Dis 2013;40(5):422–7.
51. Mavedzenge SN, Van Der Pol B, Weiss HA, et al. The association between Mycoplasma genitalium and HIV-1 acquisition in African women. AIDS 2012;26(5):617–24.
52. Barker EK, Malekinejad M, Merai R, et al. Risk of human immunodeficiency virus acquisition among high-risk heterosexuals with nonviral sexually transmitted infections: a systematic review and meta-analysis. Sex Transm Dis 2022;49(6):383–97.
53. Napierala Mavedzenge S, Müller EE, Lewis DA, et al. Mycoplasma genitalium is associated with increased genital HIV type 1 RNA in Zimbabwean women. J Infect Dis 2015;211(9):1388–98.
54. Scholes D, Stergachis A, Heidrich FE, et al. Prevention of pelvic inflammatory disease by screening for cervical chlamydial infection. N Engl J Med 1996;334(21):1362–6.
55. Workowski KA, Bachmann LH, Chan PA, et al. Sexually transmitted infections treatment guidelines, 2021. MMWR Recomm Rep (Morb Mortal Wkly Rep) 2021;70(4):1–187.
56. Jensen JS, Cusini M, Gomberg M, et al. 2021 European guideline on the management of Mycoplasma genitalium infections. J Eur Acad Dermatol Venereol 2022;36(5):641–50.
57. Soni S, Horner P, Rayment M, et al. British Association for Sexual Health and HIV national guideline for the management of infection with *Mycoplasma genitalium*

(2018). Int J STD AIDS 2019;30(10):938–50 [published correction appears in Int J STD AIDS. 2019 Aug 12;:956462419870463].
58. Ong JJ, Bourne C, Dean JA, et al. Australian sexually transmitted infection (STI) management guidelines for use in primary care 2022 update. Sex Health 2023; 20(1):1–8.
59. Canadian sti guidelines: www.canada.ca/en/public-health/services/infectious-diseases/sexual-health-sexually-transmitted-infections/canadian-guidelines/mycoplasma-genitalium.html#Key_information.
60. Falk L, Enger M, Jensen JS. Time to eradication of Mycoplasma genitalium after antibiotic treatment in men and women. J Antimicrob Chemother 2015;70(11): 3134–40.
61. FDA diagnostic information site: www.fda.gov/medical-devices/in-vitro-diagnostics/nucleic-acid-based-tests#microbial.
62. Coorevits L, Traen A, Bingé L, et al. Identifying a consensus sample type to test for Chlamydia trachomatis, Neisseria gonorrhoeae, Mycoplasma genitalium, Trichomonas vaginalis and human papillomavirus. Clin Microbiol Infect 2018; 24(12):1328–32.
63. Waites KB, Crabb DM, Ratliff AE, et al. Latest Advances in Laboratory Detection of Mycoplasma genitalium. J Clin Microbiol 2023;61(3):e0079021.
64. Bissessor M, Tabrizi SN, Twin J, et al. Macrolide resistance and azithromycin failure in a Mycoplasma genitalium-infected cohort and response of azithromycin failures to alternative antibiotic regimens. Clin Infect Dis 2015;60(8):1228–36.
65. Jensen JS, Bradshaw CS, Tabrizi SN, et al. Azithromycin treatment failure in Mycoplasma genitalium-positive patients with nongonococcal urethritis is associated with induced macrolide resistance. Clin Infect Dis 2008;47(12):1546–53.
66. Vodstrcil LA, Plummer EL, Doyle M, et al. Combination Therapy for Mycoplasma genitalium, and New Insights Into the Utility of parC Mutant Detection to Improve Cure. Clin Infect Dis 2022;75(5):813–23.
67. Murray GL, Plummer EL, Bodiyabadu K, et al. gyrA Mutations in Mycoplasma genitalium and Their Contribution to Moxifloxacin Failure: Time for the Next Generation of Resistance-Guided Therapy. Clin Infect Dis 2023;76(12):2187–95.
68. Schwebke JR, Rompalo A, Taylor S, et al. Re-evaluating the treatment of nongonococcal urethritis: emphasizing emerging pathogens–a randomized clinical trial. Clin Infect Dis 2011;52(2):163–70.
69. Mena LA, Mroczkowski TF, Nsuami M, et al. A randomized comparison of azithromycin and doxycycline for the treatment of Mycoplasma genitalium-positive urethritis in men. Clin Infect Dis 2009;48(12):1649–54.
70. Wood GE, Jensen NL, Astete S, et al. Azithromycin and Doxycycline Resistance Profiles of U.S. Mycoplasma genitalium Strains and Their Association with Treatment Outcomes. J Clin Microbiol 2021;59(11):e0081921.
71. Lau A, Bradshaw CS, Lewis D, et al. The efficacy of azithromycin for the treatment of genital mycoplasma genitalium: a systematic review and meta-analysis. Clin Infect Dis 2015;61(9):1389–99.
72. Jensen JS, Bradshaw C. Management of Mycoplasma genitalium infections - can we hit a moving target? BMC Infect Dis 2015;15:343.
73. Manhart LE, Jensen JS, Bradshaw CS, et al. Efficacy of Antimicrobial Therapy for Mycoplasma genitalium Infections. Clin Infect Dis 2015;61(Suppl 8):S802–17.
74. Machalek DA, Tao Y, Shilling H, et al. Prevalence of mutations associated with resistance to macrolides and fluoroquinolones in Mycoplasma genitalium: a systematic review and meta-analysis. Lancet Infect Dis 2020;20(11):1302–14.

75. Bachmann LH, Kirkcaldy RD, Geisler WM, et al. Prevalence of Mycoplasma genitalium Infection, Antimicrobial Resistance Mutations, and Symptom Resolution Following Treatment of Urethritis. Clin Infect Dis 2020;71(10):e624–32.
76. Murray GL, Bodiyabadu K, Vodstrcil LA, et al. *parC* Variants in Mycoplasma genitalium: Trends over Time and Association with Moxifloxacin Failure. Antimicrob Agents Chemother 2022;66(5):e0027822.
77. Xiao L, Waites KB, Van Der Pol B, et al. Mycoplasma genitalium Infections With Macrolide and Fluoroquinolone Resistance-Associated Mutations in Heterosexual African American Couples in Alabama. Sex Transm Dis 2019;46(1):18–24.
78. Dionne-Odom J, Geisler WM, Aaron KJ, et al. High Prevalence of Multidrug-Resistant Mycoplasma genitalium in Human Immunodeficiency Virus-Infected Men Who Have Sex With Men in Alabama. Clin Infect Dis 2018;66(5):796–8.
79. Ando N, Mizushima D, Takano M, et al. High prevalence of circulating dual-class resistant *Mycoplasma genitalium* in asymptomatic MSM in Tokyo, Japan. JAC Antimicrob Resist 2021;3(2):dlab091.
80. Li Y, Su X, Le W, et al. Mycoplasma genitalium in Symptomatic Male Urethritis: Macrolide Use Is Associated With Increased Resistance. Clin Infect Dis 2020; 70(5):805–10.
81. Li Y, Le WJ, Li S, et al. Meta-analysis of the efficacy of moxifloxacin in treating Mycoplasma genitalium infection. Int J STD AIDS 2017;28(11):1106–14.
82. Read TRH, Fairley CK, Murray GL, et al. Outcomes of Resistance-guided Sequential Treatment of Mycoplasma genitalium Infections: A Prospective Evaluation. Clin Infect Dis 2019;68(4):554–60.
83. Durukan D, Read TRH, Murray G, et al. Resistance-Guided Antimicrobial Therapy Using Doxycycline-Moxifloxacin and Doxycycline-2.5 g Azithromycin for the Treatment of Mycoplasma genitalium Infection: Efficacy and Tolerability. Clin Infect Dis 2020;71(6):1461–8.
84. Doyle M, Vodstrcil LA, Plummer EL, et al. Nonquinolone Options for the Treatment of *Mycoplasma genitalium* in the Era of Increased Resistance. Open Forum Infect Dis 2020;7(8):ofaa291.
85. Waites KB, Crabb DM, Atkinson TP, et al. Omadacycline Is Highly Active *In Vitro* against Mycoplasma genitalium. Microbiol Spectr 2022;10(6):e0365422.
86. Paukner S, Gruss A, Jensen JS. *In Vitro* Activity of lefamulin against sexually transmitted bacterial pathogens. Antimicrob Agents Chemother 2018;62(5): 02380.
87. Wood GE, Kim CM, Aguila LKT, et al. *In Vitro* Susceptibility and Resistance of Mycoplasma genitalium to Nitroimidazoles. Antimicrob Agents Chemother 2023; 67(4):e0000623.
88. Read TRH, Jensen JS, Fairley CK, et al. Use of Pristinamycin for Macrolide-Resistant Mycoplasma genitalium Infection. Emerg Infect Dis 2018;24(2):328–35.
89. Durukan D, Doyle M, Murray G, et al. Doxycycline and Sitafloxacin Combination Therapy for Treating Highly Resistant Mycoplasma genitalium. Emerg Infect Dis 2020;26(8):1870–4.
90. Khosropour CM, Jensen JS, Soge OO, et al. High Prevalence of Vaginal and Rectal Mycoplasma genitalium Macrolide Resistance Among Female Sexually Transmitted Disease Clinic Patients in Seattle, Washington. Sex Transm Dis 2020;47(5):321–5.
91. Sweeney EL, Whiley DM, Murray GL, et al. *Mycoplasma genitalium*: enhanced management using expanded resistance-guided treatment strategies. Sex Health 2022;19(4):248–54.

Herpes Simplex Virus

A Practical Guide to Diagnosis, Management, and Patient Counseling for the Primary Care Clinician

Teresa A. Batteiger, MD, MS[a,*], Cornelis A. Rietmeijer, MD, PhD[b]

KEYWORDS

- Herpes simplex virus (HSV) • HSV diagnosis • HSV treatment • HSV counseling

KEY POINTS

- Genital herpes is a very common sexually transmitted infection caused by herpes simplex virus (HSV)-1 or HSV-2.
- Counseling is an important aspect of the management of genital herpes.
- Transmission occurs via sexual contact; the virus can also be transmitted from mother to child during pregnancy or delivery resulting in neonatal herpes infection.
- Molecular virologic tests performed on lesions are the preferred mode of diagnosis. Serologic testing can be considered in selected cases based on the clinical scenario.
- Options for treatment of genital herpes include acyclovir, valacyclovir, and famciclovir. The duration of therapy for primary infection is longer than for recurrent outbreaks. Suppressive therapy can be used to decrease frequency of outbreaks and decrease risk of transmission.

INTRODUCTION

Genital herpes is a chronic, lifelong sexually transmitted viral infection, which can cause recurrent, self-limited genital ulcers. It is caused by herpes simplex virus (HSV) type 1 and type 2 viruses. HSV-1 can cause both oral and genital infection but is mostly associated with oral lesions (herpes labialis). HSV-2 is the leading cause of genital ulcer disease and increases risk for HIV acquisition two- to threefold.[1] Although it can cause oral lesions in rare instances, HSV-2 almost exclusively causes genital infections and is more commonly associated with recurrent outbreaks.[2,3] Most of the people infected with genital herpes are unaware of their status.[4] A National

[a] Indiana University School of Medicine, Indianapolis, IN, USA; [b] 533 Marion Street. Denver, CO 80218, USA
* Corresponding author. 1481 West 10th Street, Mail Stop 111, Indianapolis, IN 46202.
E-mail address: tbatteig@iu.edu

Med Clin N Am 108 (2024) 311–323
https://doi.org/10.1016/j.mcna.2023.08.016
0025-7125/24/Published by Elsevier Inc.
medical.theclinics.com

Health and Nutrition Examination Survey (NHANES) found that only around 13% of HSV-2 seropositive individuals had been diagnosed with genital herpes.[5] However, these individuals can still shed virus intermittently. Genital HSV is commonly encountered by primary care clinicians. Here, the authors review epidemiology, diagnosis, and management of genital herpes, illustrated by clinical vignettes and focusing on common patient questions.

Vignette 1: Transmission of Herpes Simplex Virus

A 19-year-old man presents to his primary care provider (PCP)'s office for follow-up after receiving a new diagnosis of genital HSV-1 infection, which was confirmed via type-specific nucleic acid amplification test (NAAT) of penile lesions. He does not understand how he could have acquired genital herpes because he and his female partner are monogamous and have never engaged in vaginal–penile contact. They do engage in condomless oral sex, and he notes that his partner intermittently has oral "cold sores." What is the most likely explanation?

HERPES SIMPLEX VIRUS-1 AND -2 PREVALENCE/INCIDENCE AND TRANSMISSION

Genital herpes is a common infection. In 2016, an estimated 3.7 billion people (~66.6% of the world's population under the age of 50 years) have HSV-1 infection at any site. One hundred ninety-two million people ages 15 to 49 years (prevalence of 5.2%) had genital HSV-1 infection, which accounts for ~30% of all genital infections. In addition, an estimated 491 million people (~13% of the world's population ages 15–49 years) have HSV-2 infection.[6] In the United States, Spicknall and colleagues used HSV-2 seroprevalence data from the NHANES and the American Community Survey data to obtain recent estimates. In the United States, in 2018, it was estimated that there were 572,000 incident and 18.6 million prevalent genital herpes infections among 18 to 49 year olds, with women accounting for two-thirds of the prevalent infections.[7] However, an increasing numbers of genital infections are caused by HSV-1, so the prevalence is likely higher.[8]

Both HSV-1 and HSV-2 are transmitted through sexual contact (skin and mucosal surfaces). HSV-1 can be transmitted through oral or genital sex to the partner's oral or genital areas. HSV-2 is generally transmitted from genital tract to genital tract, although genital-oral transmission occurs in rare instances. Oral HSV-1 infection does not protect against HSV-2 acquisition, but does decrease the risk for symptomatic primary genital HSV-2 infection.[9] HSV-2 infection protects against HSV-1 acquisition.[10] Because individuals can shed HSV even when asymptomatic, a significant proportion of transmission may occur from asymptomatic partners.

Vignette 1 Follow-Up: It Is Possible the Patient in Vignette 1 Could Have Acquired Genital Herpes Simplex Virus-1 from Oral-Penile Contact with His Partner

Neonatal HSV transmission happens when HSV-1 or HSV-2 exposure occurs in utero, peripartum, or postpartum. Approximately 5% of neonatal HSV is accounted for by in utero transmission. Peripartum transmission is the most common route for neonatal HSV infection. Postpartum infection occurs when the infant is exposed to orolabial or cutaneous lesions.[11] The highest risk for transmission to the neonate occurs when primary HSV infection occurs during pregnancy.[12] The risk of transmission from mother to infant is 30% to 50% in women who acquire genital herpes near the time of delivery, compared with less than 1% in women with prenatal history of recurrent genital herpes or who acquire genital herpes in the first half of pregnancy.[12,13]

Vignette 2: Clinical Manifestations and Diagnosis of Herpes Simplex Virus Infection

A 23-year-old woman comes to her PCP's office for evaluation because she has been having significant vaginal/vulvar pain and dysuria accompanied by subjective fever and malaise for the past 3 days. She denies prior history of similar symptoms. She reports a new male partner in the last month and reports condomless receptive vaginal sex. She denies oral or anal sex. On examination, she has multiple painful shallow erosions over part of the vagina and vulva. What tests should be obtained?

CLINICAL MANIFESTATIONS OF HERPES SIMPLEX VIRUS

Primary Infection

Clinical manifestations usually occur within a week of exposure. Genital symptoms classically include painful lesions but can also include dysuria, pruritus, vaginal or urethral discharge, and painful inguinal lymphadenopathy.[14] Typically, lesions start as papules or vesicles which spread rapidly over the genital area and may coalesce into larger areas of ulceration. Crusting occurs on non-mucosal surfaces, but not on mucosal surfaces.[15] Genital lesions can be unilateral or bilateral and may be extensive. In addition, systemic symptoms may occur early in the course of primary infection, including fever, headache, malaise, and myalgias.[14,15] The resolution of genital lesions occurs within 2 to 3 weeks even without antiviral therapy.[14]

Primary HSV infection can also result in urethritis, cervicitis, vulvovaginitis, and proctitis. Symptoms of urethritis associated with HSV include dysuria, meatitis, urethral discharge, and lymphadenopathy. However, in approximately 30% of cases, genital lesions are not present.[16,17] HSV-associated cervicitis is characterized by areas of focal or diffuse friability, erythema, erosive, and ulcerative lesions on the cervix with or without external herpetic lesions.[15] Primary herpes in the vagina can lead to extensive swelling, discharge, and severe dysuria. Some individuals with severe primary genital herpes outbreaks can develop urinary retention secondary to sacral radiculopathy. This is an uncommon complication, which is usually self-limited, but may require bladder catheterization until it resolves.[15,18] HSV-associated proctitis can present with rectal pain, bloody and/or mucoid discharge, and tenesmus.[15,19,20] In addition, HSV proctitis can be associated with systemic symptoms including fever, malaise, and myalgia.[15] Anal ulcerations are present in a minority of individuals.[20]

Meningitis and encephalitis are rare but may be associated with HSV infection. HSV-1 is more commonly associated with encephalitis, whereas HSV-2 is more commonly associated with meningitis.[21] HSV-2 is also associated with benign recurrent lymphocytic meningitis (Mollaret meningitis), which is characterized by recurrent episodes of meningitis which last 3 to 7 days and resolved without neurologic sequelae.[15]

Recurrent Infection

Typically, recurrent outbreaks are milder than primary infections and are heralded by a prodrome. Prodromal symptoms include burning and tingling and precede lesion development by approximately 24 hours. Lesions in recurrences are usually unilateral and fewer when compared with the primary infection.[14] Genital lesions resolve within 1 to 2 weeks even without antiviral therapy. Recurrence frequency varies widely and is more common in HSV-2 infections compared with HSV-1 infections.[3] Typically, recurrences are more frequent during the first year after infection and decline over time.[22]

Infection During Pregnancy/Neonatal Infection

Global estimates of neonatal herpes infection incidence are 10 cases/100,000 live births.[23] Rarely, infection during pregnancy has been associated with fulminant maternal hepatitis.[10] Neonatal herpes presents within 1 to 3 weeks after birth. Clinical manifestations of neonatal HSV include localized skin, eye, and mucous membrane disease (45%); central nervous system (CNS) disease (30%); and disseminated disease (25%).[24] Skin, eye and mucous membrane disease presents as vesicles and ulcers. Systemic symptoms are similar in skin, eye, and mucous membrane disease and CNS disease, which include lethargy, poor oral intake, irritability, and temperature instability. CNS disease may cause seizures. Approximately two-thirds of infants with CNS disease will have cutaneous lesions.[11] Disseminated disease presents as sepsis syndrome, respiratory distress/failure, severe liver dysfunction/failure, and disseminated intravascular coagulopathy.[25] Despite advances in diagnosis, treatment, and prevention, neonatal HSV infection continues to cause significant morbidity and mortality. Without antiviral therapy, mortality rate is estimated at 60%.[26] With antiviral therapy, mortality rates have been reported at 6% to 8% (**Box 1**).[25,27]

DIAGNOSIS OF GENITAL HERPES SIMPLEX VIRUS

Clinical diagnosis of genital herpes can be challenging as the classic lesions associated with genital herpes may have resolved or be resolving at the time of evaluation. However, if genital lesions are present at any stage, type-specific virologic testing ideally by NAAT should be performed to confirm clinical diagnosis.

Virologic Tests

HSV NAAT assays and HSV cultures can be performed on samples collected from cutaneous or mucocutaneous lesions. If vesicles or pustules are present, lesions should be unroofed and the base of the ulcer swabbed to obtain adequate cells.[28] HSV culture is generally available, but the sensitivity can be fourfold lower than HSV NAATs particularly if lesions are old and viral load is low.[29] NAATs are highly sensitive and specific and are the preferred method of testing.[30]

Serology

Serologic tests assess for antibodies to HSV. The utilization and interpretation of serologic tests for genital herpes depends on the clinical scenario. Evaluation should include history and physical examination followed by choice of appropriate diagnostic testing. The diagnosis of genital herpes by using only type-specific antibody tests can be problematic. HSV immunoglobulin M (IgM) antibodies do not distinguish between primary infection and recurrent infections and are advised against.[31,32] There are

Box 1
Differential Diagnosis of Genital Ulcers

- Syphilis (caused by *Treponema pallidum*)
- Chancroid (caused by *Haemophilus ducreyi*)
- Granuloma inguinale (caused by *Klebsiella granulomatis*)
- Lymphogranuloma venereum (caused by *Chlamydia trachomatis* serovars L1–3)
- Epstein–Barr virus
- Mpox
- Beçhet disease
- Neoplasm
- Trauma

several type-specific immunoglobulin G (IgG) assays that are commercially available for use. The type-specific IgG assays have sensitivity between 80% and 98%. Both false-negative and false-positive tests can occur. False-negative testing more frequently occur in early infection, so if there is concern for recent acquisition, repeat testing with type-specific antibody assays can be performed approximately 12 weeks following presumed time of exposure.[33–35] False-positive enzyme immunoassays occur at low index values (<3.0).[36] There is poor specificity at low index values, so confirmatory testing with a second method (ie, Western blot) should be performed before interpretation and may improve accuracy.[32] If confirmatory testing is not available, patients need to be counseled on the limitations of serologic testing and providers must be aware that false-positive tests occur.

HSV type-specific serologic testing is not recommended for:

- Screening in the general population[4,37]
- Routine screening of asymptomatic pregnant women[38]
- HSV-1 serologic screening for the diagnosis of genital HSV-1. Ideally, genital HSV-1 infection should be diagnosed by use of virologic testing (NAAT or culture).[4,39]

HSV type-specific serologic assays can be considered for:[4]

- Recurrent or atypical genital symptoms or lesions with negative virologic testing
- Clinical diagnosis of genital herpes without laboratory confirmation
- A patient whose partner was diagnosed with genital herpes.

Vignette 2 Follow-up: Primary genital HSV infection should be suspected in this patient

The following test specific to herpes should be sent: HSV NAAT from swabs from the vaginal or vulvar lesions. Additional workup might include screening for other STIs, including HIV, syphilis, gonorrhea, chlamydia.

Vignette 3: Herpes Simplex Virus Recurrence and Prevention

A 28-year-old woman has had three outbreaks of genital HSV-2 infection in the last year. She has not been sexually active for over a year. These episodes are quite painful and cause significant disruption to her life. She is wondering what her options are to manage or reduce these episodes as well as to prevent transmission to future partners. How would you counsel her?

MANAGEMENT AND TREATMENT

Acyclovir, valacyclovir, and famciclovir are approved to treat and suppress genital herpes and prevent transmission. All of these medications have excellent safety profiles.[40] There is no cure for genital herpes, but the use of antiviral medications decreases the duration of symptoms and viral shedding in both initial infection and recurrence.[41,42] **Table 1** outlines the recommended treatment regimens for genital herpes for the general population, people living with HIV, and pregnant people. Treatment of first episode should be started empirically and continued for 7 to 10 days.[4] For treatment of recurrences, dosing is higher and duration is shorter.[4,43] Antivirals should be started during the prodrome in recurrences for best outcomes.

Recurrence rates are decreased by 70% to 80% with suppressive therapy, which also reduces HSV-2 transmission among heterosexual serodiscordant partners, and should be discussed with all patients with symptomatic HSV-2 infection.[10,44–48] It should be noted that the data are limited with regard to decreasing transmission in asymptomatic patients with genital HSV-2 infection and those with genital HSV-1 infection.[4] Patients

Table 1
Recommended regimens for treatment and suppression of genital herpes

	General Population	People Living with HIV	Pregnant People
Initial infection therapy[a]			
Acyclovir	400 mg PO 3 times/day for 7–10 d	400 mg PO 3 times/day for 7–10 d	400 mg PO 3 times/day for 7–10 d
Valacyclovir	1 g PO 2 times/day for 7–10 d	1g PO 2 times/day for 7–10 d	1 g PO 2 times/day for 7–10 d
Famciclovir	250 mg PO 3 times/day for 7–10 d	250 mg PO 3 times/day for 7–10 d	
Episodic therapy			
Acyclovir	800 mg PO 2 times/day for 5 d OR 800 mg PO 3 times/day for 2 d	400 mg PO 3 times/day for 5–10 d	400 mg PO 3 times/day for 5 d OR 800 mg PO 2 times/day for 5 d
Valacyclovir	500 mg PO 2 times/day for 3 d OR 1g PO daily for 5 d	1 g PO 2 times/day for 5–10 d	500 mg PO 2 times/day for 3 d OR 1 g PO daily for 5 d
Famciclovir	1 g PO 2 times/day for 1 d OR 500 mg PO once, followed by 250 mg 2 times/day for 2 d OR 125 mg PO 2 times/day for 5 d	500 mg PO 2 times/day for 5–10 d	
Suppressive therapy[b]			
Acyclovir	400 mg PO 2 times/day	400–800 mg PO 2–3 times/day	400 mg PO 3 times/day
Valacyclovir	500 mg PO daily[c] OR 1g PO daily	500 mg PO 2 times/day	500 mg PO 2 times/day
Famciclovir	250 mg PO 2 times/day	500 mg PO 2 times/day	

[a] Treatment can be extended if healing is incomplete after 10 days of therapy.
[b] In pregnant people, suppressive therapy is recommended starting at 36 wk gestation.
[c] Valacyclovir 500 mg daily may be less effective than other valacyclovir or acyclovir dosing regimens for persons who have frequent recurrences (ie, ≥10 episodes/year).

Source: Based on CDC STI Treatment Guidelines (https://www.cdc.gov/std/treatment-guidelines/) and *Adapted from* Table 1 in Van Wagoner et al. Inf Dis Clin North Am 2023.

should be counseled on the potential for breakthrough lesions and viral shedding.[49] The continued use of suppressive therapy should be revisited periodically.[10]

Treatment in Pregnancy

All pregnant people should be asked about history of genital herpes or genital signs or symptoms concerning for genital herpes during their pregnancy and at the time of delivery. If no signs or symptoms of genital herpes, vaginal delivery is acceptable. However, if active genital lesions are present at the time of delivery, cesarean delivery is recommended to decrease the risk for neonatal HSV infection.[4,13] Acyclovir is safe in pregnancy and breastfeeding and is recommended for use in pregnant people for first episode and recurrent episodes of genital herpes.[4,50,51] For pregnant people with known history of genital herpes, the use of suppressive therapy starting at 36 weeks gestation decreased the risk for recurrent episodes of genital herpes, although break through cases of neonatal herpes have been reported.[52,53] For pregnant people who acquire HSV during pregnancy, empirical antiviral therapy is recommended while awaiting confirmation, and then, suppressive antiviral therapy is recommended starting at 36 weeks if infection occurs early in pregnancy.[4]

Treatment in People Living with Human Immunodeficiency Virus

Antiretroviral therapy (ART) and immune reconstitution are major elements of genital herpes management. Even with immune reconstitution and ART, recurrences are more frequent in people living with human immunodeficiency virus (HIV) (PLWH). In PLWH with low CD4 counts on initiation of ART (<200 cells/mm^3), frequency of recurrences increases in the first 6 months.[10] Treatment is similar to other populations, although dose and duration are increased.[4] Suppressive therapy does not reduce the risk for HIV or HSV-2 transmission in coinfected people.[54,55]

PREVENTION

There are limited options for prevention of genital herpes transmission to partners in addition to suppressive therapy. Compared with no condoms, consistent and correct condom use resulted in a 30% decreased risk of HSV-2 acquisition.[56] In another study, it was found that HSV-2 transmission protection from condom use was different by sex. Correct condom use decreased the per-act transmission risk from cis-men to cis-women by 96% and from cis-women to cis-men by 65%.[57] There are no data on impact of condom use for prevention in anal sex. In addition, there is ongoing research on developing preventive and therapeutic vaccines for prevention of transmission, but currently there is no effective vaccine available.[10]

Vignette 3 Follow-Up

This patient has two available options for management of the frequent outbreaks: episodic or suppressive therapy. Given frequency of the outbreaks and reported significant pain associated with outbreaks, suppressive therapy may be more beneficial to the patient if she is willing to take daily medication. Continued need for suppressive therapy should be reassessed periodically.

COUNSELING

Genital herpes is quite stigmatized, and patients are often distressed on receiving the diagnosis.[58,59] Patients may feel shame, guilt, or anger; distress regarding transmission; fear of partner reactions; and difficulty in disclosing status.[60] Providing counseling to the individual with genital herpes and their sex partners is an important part of the management of genital herpes.[4] The major goals of counseling include helping the patient understand the infection, options for treatment, access resources for information, and prevent sexual and perinatal transmission.[4,60]

Counseling discordant couples is particularly challenging, especially in case of committed relationships where the (cis-gender) female partner is uninfected and where future pregnancy is desired. Despite the effectiveness of suppressive treatment, avoiding sex during outbreaks, and condom use, transmission may still occur over the long term. Moreover, couples may feel that such preventive measures will interfere with their (sexual) relationship and may decide to let "nature runs its course," knowing that for the female partner, infection occurring before pregnancy is preferable over infection occurring during pregnancy, especially during the second half. An open discussion of pros and cons should be the basis of a shared decision-making process. Regardless, infection status should be determined in the early phases of pregnancy of

Table 2
Common herpes simplex virus-related patient questions/concerns: summary of counseling points[a]

Patient Question/Concern	Counseling Points
What causes genital herpes?	• Caused by a virus • There are two types of HSV (HSV-1 and HSV-2) • Both types can cause genital herpes • It is a common condition • No cure, the virus persists in the body (latent state)
I have never been diagnosed with an STI or HIV. I do not have any symptoms currently, nor do I have a history of any previous or recurrent genital symptoms. None of my sexual partners have had STIs that I know of. I am not pregnant. I want to get routine STI screening "just to be safe." Should I be tested for HSV?	• Routine screening for HSV in asymptomatic individuals is not recommended for most people • Routine screening for other STIs generally includes testing for HIV, gonorrhea, chlamydia, and syphilis • It is important to screen for gonorrhea and chlamydia at sites that are exposed during sex
How did I get genital herpes?	• Transmission occurs through skin-to-skin or mucous membrane contact • Transmission can occur even when a person is asymptomatic
Can I get genital herpes through oral sex?	• Genital HSV-1 infection can occur from receiving oral sex from a partner who has oral herpes (HSV-1) • Genital HSV-2 infection can occur through oral sex, although is rare
My partner and I have had other sexual partners in the past but have been in a monogamous relationship for the past 8 mo. I have just had an episode of genital ulcers for the first time and was diagnosed with genital herpes. Does this mean my partner has definitely had other partners in the past 8 mo they are not telling me about?	• Many people infected with genital herpes are unaware of their status • Intermittent viral shedding can occur in asymptomatic individuals • Transmission may occur from asymptomatic individual who may be unaware of their status • Current diagnostics do not allow for determination of timing of infection
If I have HSV 1 can I get HSV 2 (and vice versa)?	• You can have both HSV-1 and HSV-2 • Oral HSV-1 infection does not protect against HSV-2 acquisition • Oral HSV-1 does decrease the risk for symptomatic primary genital HSV-2 infection • HSV-2 infection does protect against HSV-1 acquisition
I have just been diagnosed with HSV—who do I need to tell?	• Last sexual partner, current partner, and future partners should be told. • Current partners should be informed and receive testing.

(*continued on next page*)

Table 2
(*continued*)

Patient Question/Concern	Counseling Points
How can I avoid giving my future partners HSV?	• Avoid sex during prodrome/outbreak • Condoms reduce but do not eliminate transmission • Suppressive therapy reduces but does not eliminate transmission • Risk for transmission increases during outbreaks • Individuals with genital herpes can have healthy sex lives
I am worried about how my partner will react to the news of my HSV diagnosis—what can I do?	• Support group availability • Individual or couples counseling
I feel very guilty and ashamed about this diagnosis—what can I do?	• Sex is normal and important part of life • Genital herpes is very common • Suppressive therapy helps decrease frequency of outbreaks • Support groups are available
Does having HSV mean I cannot get pregnant or that if I do it will harm the baby?	• Fertility not affected • Does not prevent an individual from having children • Routine screening for HSV not recommended during pregnancy • If partner is known to have genital herpes and pregnant person has no known history of genital herpes, type-specific serologic tests for the pregnant person can be helpful for counseling • Suppressive therapy starting at 36 wk gestation decreases risk of viral shedding during delivery in those with recurrent genital herpes
I am pregnant at 14 wk, I do not have a known history of HSV but my male partner has a history of genital HSV outbreaks. What should I do?	• Highest risk for neonatal herpes is when a woman becomes infected late in pregnancy • Women with no history of genital herpes should abstain from sex with partners known or suspected to have genital herpes in the third trimester • Women with no known history of orolabial herpes should abstain from receptive oral sex with partners known to have or suspected to have orolabial herpes in the third trimester. • Type-specific serologic tests can be useful for guiding counseling (see above).
Other concerns	• Genital herpes is a manageable condition • Treatment of outbreaks with safe and effective antivirals • Genital herpes does not cause cancer • Genital herpes can increase risk for acquiring HIV infection (counseling on pre-exposure prophylaxis (PrEP))

[a] See also Table 2 in Van Wagoner et al. Inf Dis Clin North Am 2023.

any woman in a discordant relationship to prevent the possibility of vertical transmission and its devastating sequelae.

Table 2 outlines the key points to address with regard to frequently encountered patient concerns/questions. The Centers for Disease Control and Prevention and the Canadian Government have resources for counseling tools.[4,60]

SUMMARY

Genital HSV infection is a very prevalent STI, which causes self-limited, recurrent genital ulcers. Treatment decreases duration of symptoms and signs and can be provided as episodic or suppressive therapy. Genital herpes can have a substantial impact during pregnancy and on sexual health in general. Counseling on natural history, transmission, treatment, and management of sexual partners is an integral part of management of genital herpes.

CLINICS CARE POINTS

- Nucleic acid amplification tests (NAATs) are more sensitive than culture and are the preferred method of testing for individuals with genital lesions.
- Type-specific serologic assays (IgG) can be used in certain clinical scenarios but are not recommended for screening in the general population.
- Clinical manifestations in primary infection can include genital and systemic symptoms and signs and are generally more severe than recurrent episodes.
- Antiviral therapy decreases duration of clinical manifestations and viral shedding. Suppressive therapy can decrease frequency of recurrences and reduce the risk of transmission.
- In pregnant people, acyclovir and valacyclovir should be used to treat first-episode and recurrences. Suppressive therapy with acyclovir is recommended starting at 36 weeks gestation to reduce recurrences at delivery.
- Counseling is an important aspect of the management of genital herpes as genital herpes is stigmatized and can cause substantial distress for patients.

DISCLOSURE

T.A. Batteiger and C.A. Rietmeijer have no disclosures.

REFERENCES

1. Masese L, Baeten JM, Richardson B, et al. Changes in the contribution of genital tract infections to HIV acquisition among Kenyan high-risk women from 1993 to 2012. AIDS 2015;29(9):1077–85.
2. Benedetti J, Corey L, Ashley R. Recurrence rates in genital herpes after symptomatic first-episode infection. Ann Intern Med 1994;121(11):847–54.
3. Engelberg R, Carrell D, Krantz E, et al. Natural history of genital herpes simplex virus type 1 infection. Sex Transm Dis 2003;30(2):174–7.
4. Workowski KA, Bachmann LH, Chan PA, et al. Sexually Transmitted Infections Treatment Guidelines, 2021. MMWR Recomm Rep (Morb Mortal Wkly Rep) 2021;70(4):1–187.
5. Fanfair R, Azaidi A, Taylor L, et al. Trends in seroprevlaence of herpes simplex virus type 2 among non-Hispanic blacks and non-Hispanic whites aged 14 to 49 years - United States, 1988-2010. Sex Transm Dis 2013;40:860–4.

6. James C, Harfouche M, Welton NJ, et al. Herpes simplex virus: global infection prevalence and incidence estimates, 2016. Bull World Health Organ 2020; 98(5):315–29.
7. Spicknall IH, Flagg EW, Torrone EA. Estimates of the Prevalence and Incidence of Genital Herpes, United States, 2018. Sex Transm Dis 2021;48(4):260–5.
8. McQuillan G, Kruszon-Moran D, Flagg EW, et al. Prevalence of Herpes Simplex Virus Type 1 and Type 2 in Persons Aged 14-49: United States, 2015-2016. NCHS Data Brief 2018;304(304):1–8.
9. Corey L, Holmes KK. Genital herpes simplex virus infections: current concepts in diagnosis, therapy, and prevention. Ann Intern Med 1983;98(6):973–83.
10. Van Wagoner N, Qushair F, Johnston C. Genital Herpes Infection: Progress and Problems. Infect Dis Clin North Am 2023;37(2):351–67.
11. James S, Kimberlin D. Neonatal herpes simplex virus infection. Infect Dis Clin North Am 2015;29(3):391–400.
12. Brown Z, Benedetti J, Ashley R, et al. Neonatal herpes simplex virus infection in relation to asymptomatic maternal infection at the time of labor. N Engl J Med 1991;324(18):1247–52.
13. Brown ZA, Wald A, Morrow RA, et al. Effect of serologic status and cesarean delivery on transmission rates of herpes simplex virus from mother to infant. JAMA 2003;289(2):203–9.
14. Corey L, Adams HG, Brown ZA, et al. Genital herpes simplex virus infections: clinical manifestations, course, and complications. Ann Intern Med 1983;98(6): 958–72.
15. Corey L. and Wald A., Genital Herpes, In: Holmes K., Sparling P., Stamm W., et al., editors. *Sexually transmitted diseases*, 4th edition, 2008. The McGraw-Hills Companies, Inc.: New York, 399–437, chap 24.
16. Ong J, Morton A, Henzell H, et al. Clinical characteristics of herpes simplex virus urethritis compared with chlamydial urethritis among men. Sex Transm Dis 2017; 44(2):121–5.
17. Bradshaw CS, Tabrizi SN, Read TR, et al. Etiologies of nongonococcal urethritis: bacteria, viruses, and the association with orogenital exposure. J Infect Dis 2006; 193(3):336–45.
18. Whalen AM, Mateo CM, Growdon AS, et al. Sacral Myeloradiculitis: An Uncommon Complication of Genital Herpes Infection. Pediatrics 2019;144(1). https://doi.org/10.1542/peds.2018-2631.
19. Pinto-Sander N, Parkes L, Fitzpatrick C, et al. Symptomatic sexually transmitted proctitis in men who have sex with men. Sex Transm Infect 2019;95(6):471.
20. Bissessor M, Fairley C, Read T, et al. The etiology of infectious proctitis in men who have sex with men differs according to HIV status. Sex Transm Dis 2013; 40(10):768–70.
21. Gundamraj V, Hasbun R. Viral meningitis and encephalitis: an update. Curr Opin Infect Dis 2023;36(3):177–85.
22. Benedetti JK, Zeh J, Corey L. Clinical reactivation of genital herpes simplex virus infection decreases in frequency over time. Ann Intern Med 1999;131(1):14–20.
23. Looker KJ, Magaret AS, May MT, et al. First estimates of the global and regional incidence of neonatal herpes infection. Lancet Glob Health 2017;5(3):e300–9.
24. Fernandes N, Arya K, Ward R. Congenital herpes simplex. Treasure Island (FL): StatPearls Publishing; 2023. https://www.ncbi.nlm.nih.gov/books/NBK507897/.
25. Mahant S, Hall M, Schondelmeyer A, et al. Neonatal herpes simplex virus infection among Medicaid-Enrolled Children: 2009-2015. Pediatrics 2019;143(4): e20183233.

26. Melvin AJ, Mohan KM, Vora SB, et al. Neonatal Herpes Simplex Virus Infection: Epidemiology and Outcomes in the Modern Era. J Pediatric Infect Dis Soc 2022;11(3):94–101.
27. Donda K, Sharma M, Amponsah J, et al. Trends in the incidence, mortality, and cost of neonatal herpes simplex virus hospitalizations in the United States from 2003-2014. J Perinatol 2019;39:697–707.
28. Johnston C, Corey L. Current concepts for genital herpes simplex virus infection: Diagnostics and pathogenesis of genital tract shedding. Clin Microbiol Rev 2016; 29(1):149–61.
29. Wald A, Huang ML, Carrell D, et al. Polymerase chain reaction for detection of herpes simplex virus (HSV) DNA on mucosal surfaces: comparison with HSV isolation in cell culture. J Infect Dis 2003;188(9):1345–51.
30. Strick L, Wald A. Diagnostics for herpes simplex virus: Is PCR the new gold standard? Mol Diagn Thera 2006;10(1):17–28.
31. Page J, Taylor J, Tideman R, et al. Is HSV serology useful for the management of first episode genital herpes? Sex Transm Infect 2003;79(4):276–9.
32. Morrow R, Friedrich D. Performance of a novel test for IgM and IgG antibodies in subjects with culture-documented genital herpes simplex virus-1 or -2 infection. Clin Microbiol Infect 2006;12(5):463–9.
33. Whittington W, Celum C, Cent A, et al. Use of a glycoprotein G-based type-specific assay to detect antibodies to herpes simplex virus type 2 among persons attending sexually transmitted disease clinics. Sex Transm Dis 2001;28:99–104.
34. Turner K, Wong E, Kent C, et al. Serologic herpes testing in the real world: validation of new type-specific serologic herpes simplex virus tests in a public health laboratory. Sex Transm Dis 2002;29:422–5.
35. Eing B, Lippelt L, Lorentzen E, et al. Evaluation of confirmatory strategies for detection of type-specific antibodies against herpes simplex virus type 2. J Clin Microbiol 2002;40:407–13.
36. Ngo T, Laeyendecker O, La H, et al. Use of commercial enzyme immunoassays to detect antibodies to the herpes simplex virus type 2 glycoprotein G in a low-risk population in Hanoi, Vietnam. Clin Vaccine Immunol 2008;15:382–4.
37. Feltner C, Grodensky C, Ebel C, et al. Serologic Screening for Genital Herpes: An Updated Evidence Report and Systematic Review for the US Preventive Services Task Force. JAMA 2016;316(23):2531–43.
38. Bulletins ACoP. ACOG Practice Bulletin. Clinical management guidelines for obstetrician-gynecologist. No. 82 June 2017. Management of herpes in pregnancy. Obstet Gynecol 2007;109(6):1489–98.
39. Johnston C. Diagnosis and Management of Genital Herpes: Key Questions and Review of the Evidence for the 2021 Centers for Disease Control and Prevention Sexually Transmitted Infections Treatment Guidelines. Clin Infect Dis 2022; 74(Suppl_2):S134–43.
40. Johnson RE, Mullooly JP, Valanis BG, et al. Utilization and safety of oral acyclovir over an 8-year period. Pharmacoepidemiol Drug Saf 1997;6(2):101–13.
41. Corey L, Benedetti J, Critchlow C, et al. Treatment of primary first-episode genital herpes simplex virus infections with acyclovir: results of topical, intravenous and oral therapy. J Antimicrob Chemother 1983;12(Suppl B):79–88.
42. Sacks SL, Aoki FY, Diaz-Mitoma F, et al. Patient-initiated, twice-daily oral famciclovir for early recurrent genital herpes. A randomized, double-blind multicenter trial. Canadian Famciclovir Study Group. JAMA 1996;276(1):44–9.
43. Spruance S, Aoki FY, Tyring S, et al. Short-course therapy for recurrent genital herpes and herpes labialis. J Fam Pract 2007;56(1):30–6.

44. Reitano M, Tyring S, Lang W, et al. Valacyclovir for the suppression of recurrent genital herpes virus infection: A large-scale dose range-finding study. International Valaciclovir HSV Study Group. J Infect Dis 1998;178(6):603–10.
45. Diaz-Mitoma F, Sibbald RG, Shafran SD, et al. Oral famciclovir for the suppression of recurrent genital herpes: a randomized controlled trial. Collaborative Famciclovir Genital Herpes Research Group. JAMA 1998;280(10):887–92.
46. Mertz GJ, Loveless MO, Levin MJ, et al. Oral famciclovir for suppression of recurrent genital herpes simplex virus infection in women. A multicenter, double-blind, placebo-controlled trial. Collaborative Famciclovir Genital Herpes Research Group. Arch Intern Med 1997;157(3):343–9.
47. Corey L, Wald A, Patel R, et al. Once-daily valacyclovir to reduce the risk of transmission of genital herpes. N Engl J Med 2004;350(1):11–20.
48. Patel R, Tyring S, Strand A, et al. Impact of suppressive antiviral therapy on the health related quality of life of patients with recurrent genital herpes infection. Sex Transm Infect 1999;75(6):398–402.
49. Johnston C, Saracino M, Kuntz S, et al. Standard-dose and high-dose daily antiviral therapy for short episodes of genital HSV-2 reactivation: three randomised, open-label, cross-over trials. Lancet 2012;379(9816):641–7.
50. Pasternak B, Hviid A. Use of acyclovir, valacyclovir, and famciclovir in the first trimester of pregnancy and the risk of birth defects. JAMA 2010;304(8):859–66.
51. Stone K, Reiff-Eldridge R, White A, et al. Pregnancy outcomes following systemic prenatal acyclovir exposure: Conclusions from the international acyclovir pregnancy registry, 1984-1999. Birth Defects Res A Clin Mol Teratol 2004;70(4):201–7.
52. Watts DH, Brown ZA, Money D, et al. A double-blind, randomized, placebo-controlled trial of acyclovir in late pregnancy for the reduction of herpes simplex virus shedding and cesarean delivery. Am J Obstet Gynecol 2003;188(3):836–43.
53. Marrazzo J, Rabe L, Kelly C, et al. Tenofovir gel for prevention of herpes simplex virus type 2 acquisition: Findings from the VOICE Trial. J Infect Dis 2019;219(12): 1940–7.
54. Mujugira A, Magaret AS, Celum C, et al. Daily acyclovir to decrease herpes simplex virus type 2 (HSV-2) transmission from HSV-2/HIV-1 coinfected persons: a randomized controlled trial. J Infect Dis 2013;208(9):1366–74.
55. Celum C, Wald A, Lingappa JR, et al. Acyclovir and transmission of HIV-1 from persons infected with HIV-1 and HSV-2. N Engl J Med 2010;362(5):427–39.
56. Martin ET, Krantz E, Gottlieb SL, et al. A pooled analysis of the effect of condoms in preventing HSV-2 acquisition. Arch Intern Med 2009;169(13):1233–40.
57. Magaret AS, Mujugira A, Hughes JP, et al. Effect of Condom Use on Per-act HSV-2 Transmission Risk in HIV-1, HSV-2-discordant Couples. Clin Infect Dis 2016; 62(4):456–61.
58. Melville J, Sniffen S, Crosby R, et al. Psychosocial impact of serological diagnosis of herpes simplex virus type 2: a qualitative assessment. Sex Transm Infect 2003; 79(4):280–5.
59. Romanowski B, Zdanowicz YM, Owens ST. In search of optimal genital herpes management and standard of care (INSIGHTS): doctors' and patients' perceptions of genital herpes. Sex Transm Infect 2008;84(1):51–6.
60. Steben M, Fisher M. Genital herpes counselling tool. Government of Canada. Updated March 8, 2019. Available at: https://www.canada.ca/en/public-health/services/infectious-diseases/sexual-health-sexually-transmitted-infections/canadian-guidelines/sexually-transmitted-infections/genital-herpes-counselling-tool.html. Accessed June 14, 2023.

Syphilis Serologies

A Practical Approach for the Primary Care Clinician

Elizabeth A. Gilliams, MD, MSc[a,*], Zachary Lorenz, MD[b], Matthew M. Hamill, MBChB, PhD[a]

KEYWORDS

- Syphilis • Serology • Sexually transmitted infection • Treponemal testing

KEY POINTS

- Diagnosis of syphilis relies on reactive treponemal-specific and non-treponemal antibody testing and clinical assessment. Local health departments can often provide a syphilis testing and treatment history.
- Serologic antibody testing may be nonreactive early in infection, leading to false-negative results.
- Ensure adequate time has passed (12 months for primary and secondary syphilis, 24 months for latent syphilis) before making a decision about serologic treatment success.
- Lumbar puncture is only indicated in specific scenarios, such as when a patient has neurologic symptoms or non-treponemal test titers increase ≥4-fold in the absence of reexposure.
- Remember to test for HIV and offer HIV pre-exposure prophylaxis to patients with syphilis.

INTRODUCTION

Syphilis is a sexually transmitted infection (STI) caused by *Treponema pallidum* (TP). In 2021, the Centers for Disease Control and Prevention (CDC) reported 176,213 cases of syphilis, a 74% increase since 2017.[1] Although men who have sex with men accounted for almost half (46%) of all primary and secondary syphilis cases, a sustained epidemic among the heterosexual population has also been observed. Paralleling increases in cases among reproductive-aged women, congenital syphilis (CS) cases have

[a] Division of Infectious Diseases, Johns Hopkins University School of Medicine, Johns Hopkins Bayview Medical Center, 5200 Eastern Avenue, Baltimore, MD 21224, USA; [b] Department of Medicine, Johns Hopkins University School of Medicine, Johns Hopkins Bayview Medical Center, Baltimore, MD 21224, USA

* Corresponding author. Division of Infectious Diseases, Johns Hopkins University School of Medicine, Johns Hopkins Bayview Medical Center, Mason F. Lord Center Tower, Suite 381, 5200 Eastern Avenue, Baltimore, MD 21224.

E-mail address: Egillia8@jhmi.edu

Med Clin N Am 108 (2024) 325–337
https://doi.org/10.1016/j.mcna.2023.08.002
medical.theclinics.com

increased. In 2021, the national CS rate was 77.9 cases per 100,000 live births; a 219.3% increase relative to 2017. Syphilis stages, serologic profiles, and treatment recommendations are reviewed in **Table 1**.

The direct identification of TP (eg, polymerase chain reaction [PCR], dark-field microscopy) is possible but not widely available. Serology is the most common, indirect, diagnostic test for syphilis. Syphilis serology is classified into treponemal tests (TTs; eg, TP passive particle agglutination assay [TP-PA], FTA-ABS [fluorescent treponemal antibody absorption]) and non-treponemal tests (NTTs; eg, RPR [rapid plasma reagin] and VDRL [veneral disease research laboratory]). **Fig. 1** displays a full list of assays. TTs and NTTs differ by their antigen target. TTs detect antibody to TP proteins, whereas NTTs detect nonspecific antibodies directed against lipoidal antigens, damaged host cells, and treponemes.[4]

Two-stage serologic testing with a TT and NTT, along with clinical staging, is required to make a syphilis diagnosis. It is crucial that a provider know the testing algorithm used by their institution or practice. The traditional (or standard) algorithm uses an NTT and reflexes to a TT if reactive, whereas the reverse algorithm begins with a TT and reflexes to an NTT if reactive (see **Fig. 1**). In the case of discordant TT and NTT in the reverse algorithm a second, different, TT is used as a "tiebreaker." There are key principles of syphilis serologies which can be useful to the clinician in navigating their nuances.

The first principle is that TTs generally remain reactive for life (in at least 75% of individuals after initial infection), regardless of treatment.[5] TTs provide no insight as to when a patient was infected, if treatment was completed, or if reinfection has occurred. A reactive TT alone should not necessarily prompt treatment for syphilis, but rather further investigation.

The second key principle is that NTTs offer dilutional antibody titers (eg, 1:64). NTTs are clinically useful in monitoring response to treatment and in distinguishing reinfection from old previously treated infection. NTTs may become nonreactive in persons who are treated for syphilis but also can decline over time in the absence of treatment. The reverse algorithm is more sensitive in detecting prior syphilis infection. In primary syphilis, TTs have sensitivities between 82% and 100%,[4] exceeding those of NTTs with sensitivities between 62% and 76%.[6]

Syphilis serology testing has specific pitfalls that are important for the clinician to be aware of. The goal of this review is to describe a series of clinical scenarios that demonstrate the challenges of syphilis serologic interpretation and provide a rationale for management.

Vignette 1: Primary Syphilis

A 43-year-old man contacts his primary care provider requesting testing for STIs and citing the appearance of a painless lesion on his penis 2 days earlier. Six weeks before the lesion appearing, he had condomless oral and anal-receptive intercourse with two new male partners. He was previously in a monogamous relationship and has never had an STI. He is offered empirical treatment for primary syphilis with a single intramuscular injection of 2.4 million international units (MIU) of benzathine penicillin G [BPG] but declines. Specimens sent for testing on the day of initial presentation for *Chlamydia trachomatis*, *Neisseria gonorrhea*, HIV, and herpes simplex virus were all unrevealing, including nonreactive TP enzyme immunoassay (TP-EIA) and RPR. The patient is informed and again offered empirical treatment for primary syphilis, but prefers to return for repeat testing 2 weeks later. His lesion has resolved, and he has no penile discharge, fever, sore throat, rash, or lymphadenopathy. Repeat testing is obtained and notable for a reactive TP-EIA with an RPR antibody titer of 1:32.

Table 1
Stages of syphilis, typical clinical features, expected serologic status, and recommended treatment regimens per 2021 CDC Sexually Transmitted Infection Treatment Guidelines

Stage	Typical Clinical Features	Serology[2]	Treatment[3]
Primary	Painless ulcer (chancre)	TT and NTT may be nonreactive in up to 30%	Recommended: BPG 2.4 MIU once IM Alternative: Doxycycline 100 mg BID for 14 d[a]
Secondary	Any part of the body can be affected. Typical rash is truncal, with palms and soles involved	TT and NTT tests are reactive	Recommended: BPG 2.4 MIU once IM Alternative: Doxycycline 100 mg BID for 14 d[a]
Early latent (<1 y)	No signs or symptoms	TT reactive NTT may be reactive or nonreactive	Recommended: BPG 2.4 MIU once IM Alternative: Doxycycline 100 mg BID for 14 d[a]
Late latent (≥1 y) or Unknown duration			Recommended: BPG 2.4 MIU IM on days 0, 7, 14, for a total of 7.2 MIU Alternative: Doxycycline 100 mg BID for 28 d[a]
Tertiary • Cardiac • Gummatous	Depends on location of lesion(s)	TT reactive NTT may be reactive or nonreactive	Depends on CSF result. If positive, treat for neurologic syphilis. If negative CSF, BPG 2.4 MIU IM on days 0, 7, 14, for a total of 7.2 MIU
Neurologic • Early	Headache, stroke, cranial nerve palsies	TT reactive NTT typically reactive	Recommended: Parenteral aqueous penicillin G 18–24 MIU per day, administered as 3–4 MIU IV every 4 h or continuous infusion for 10–14 d Alternative: Procaine penicillin 2.4 MIU IM once daily, PLUS Probenecid 500 mg orally 4 times/day, both for 10–14 d Ceftriaxone 1–2 g daily either IM or IV for 10–14 d (limited data)[a]
Neurologic • Late	Meningovascular: strokes Parenchymatous: (tabes and general paresis) Tabes: shooting pain in the back; gait abnormalities General paresis: cognitive declines (dementia); personality changes; hallucinations	TT reactive NTT typically reactive (NTT uncommonly nonreactive)	
Neurologic • Ocular • Otic	Ocular: Uveitis, neuroretinitis, optic neuritis Otic: Hearing loss, tinnitus	TT reactive NTT typically reactive (NTT uncommonly nonreactive)	

TT, treponemal test; NTT, non-treponemal test; BPG, benzathine penicillin G; MIU, million international units; BID, twice daily; CSF, cerebrospinal fluid; IV, intravenous; IM, intramuscular.
[a] Thorough clinical and serologic follow-up of persons receiving any alternative therapy is essential.

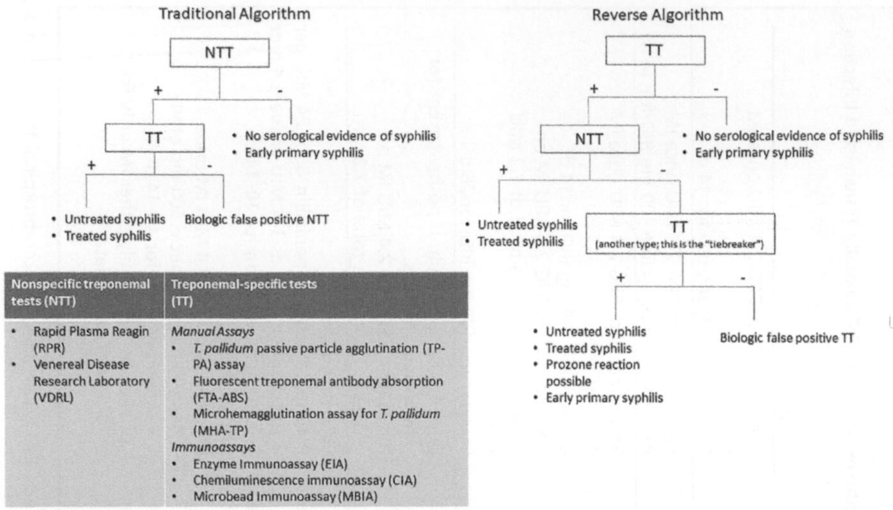

Fig. 1. Description of the traditional and reverse testing algorithms and their interpretations.

Discussion

Primary syphilis is heralded by a genital papule which quickly blossoms to a localized and indurated, usually painless ulcer (chancre) with raised margins at the point of inoculation. The median incubation period for a chancre is approximately 21 days and can develop as late as 3 months after exposure.[7] Alternatively, chancres may be multiple, painful, and found at any site of sexual contact including oropharynx, rectum, and cervix.[8] Chancres, when painless, may go unnoticed by the patient. Providers should consider primary syphilis in the differential diagnosis of genital ulcer disease including herpetic lesions, mpox, hemorrhoids, malignancies, inflammatory bowel disease, and other infections. Even in the absence of treatment, chancres resolve within 3 to 6 weeks.[7]

This case provides a key lesson: all serologic assays (TTs and NTTs) can be falsely negative in early disease.[6] This is usually because the test was obtained before TP antibody formation has occurred but can also reflect a rare phenomenon termed the prozone effect. The prozone effect occurs when an excess of antibodies interferes with the visualization of agglutination of an antibody-antigen complex and is more common in primary and secondary syphilis.[6] If there is high clinical suspicion for syphilis, the clinician can notify the laboratory of a suspected prozone effect and request additional dilutions and repeat testing of the sample. For patients in whom there is a high clinical suspicion for primary syphilis, empirical therapy should also be considered.

This patient initially had seronegative primary syphilis, with nonreactive syphilis serologies at the time of their chancre. Seronegative primary syphilis is a well-characterized phenomenon that occurs in up to 30% of patients.[6] It is more prone to occur via the traditional algorithm because TT tends to become reactive before NTTs but can occur with either algorithm.[9] Providers may opt to treat chancres presumptively, pending the result of serologic tests; this will depend on sexual history and epidemiologic risk factors. In individuals with evidence of primary syphilis and who have nonreactive syphilis serologies, testing should be repeated in 2 weeks.[10]

Vignette 2: Secondary Syphilis

A 19-year-old man presents to the emergency department with a 5-day history of worsening fever, myalgias, and rash. He has no significant medical history, is up to date with immunizations, and is not taking any medications. On examination, his temperature is 37.6°C, he has no evidence of meningismus or nuchal rigidity, and neurologic examination is normal. He has sub-centimeter lymphadenopathy in the inguinal, axillary, and epitrochlear regions. A widespread, papular rash is evident on the chest, torso, and back; his palms and soles are not involved. He identifies as bisexual, has condomless sex with male and female partners and is not taking HIV pre-exposure prophylaxis (PrEP). His last sexual exposure was 6 weeks ago, during which he had receptive anal sex with a male he met online. Acute HIV, Epstein Barr Virus (EBV), and syphilis are considered in the differential diagnosis. HIV antigen/antibody test, HIV ribonucleic acid (RNA) assay, and EBV serology were nonreactive or undetectable. However, TP-EIA is positive and a reflex RPR is reactive with a titer of 1:128.

He is diagnosed with secondary syphilis, treated with a single dose of BPG 2.4 MIU intramuscularly and discharged with follow-up for initiation of PrEP given this recent diagnosis of syphilis. At 1 month follow-up, he begins daily PrEP with tenofovir disoproxil fumarate/emtricitabine, and at a 3 month follow-up visit, the RPR titer has declined to 1:64 (a twofold/one-dilution decrease). He subsequently misses his 6 month follow-up visit, but at 12 months, his HIV tests remain negative and the RPR titer is now 1:4 (**Fig. 2**), representing a 32-fold decrease from its peak.

Discussion

Successful treatment of primary or secondary syphilis is defined by resolution of signs and symptoms and by at least a fourfold decline in RPR titer, for example, from an initial titer of 1:128 to 1:32 (**Fig. 3**). CDC guidelines recommend repeat RPR titers at 6 and 12 months but waiting a full 12 months after treatment of primary and secondary syphilis (24 months in those with HIV) before adjudication of treatment success (see **Fig. 2**). In the absence of evidence of reexposure, providers should allow the full recommended time to elapse before considering treatment failure. A $\geq$ 4-fold increase in RPR titer at any time following treatment that is sustained when repeated after a minimum of 2 weeks should prompt an evaluation for reinfection or treatment failure.

Patients often find it difficult to recall their RPR titers. This can pose a challenge when they change providers and particularly if they move between states or countries.

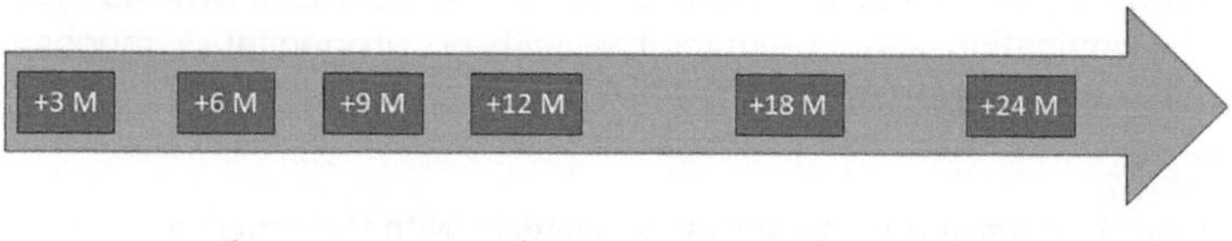

	+3 M	+6 M	+9 M	+12 M	+18 M	+24 M
Primary and Secondary Syphilis[a]		✓		✓		
Primary and Secondary Syphilis (PWH)	✓	✓	✓	✓		✓
Latent syphilis (early and late)		✓		✓		✓
Latent syphilis (early and late- PWH)		✓		✓	✓	✓

Fig. 2. CDC recommended stage-specific posttreatment intervals for follow-up. NTT, nontreponemal test; PWH, persons with HIV; M, months. [a] Consider more frequent testing.

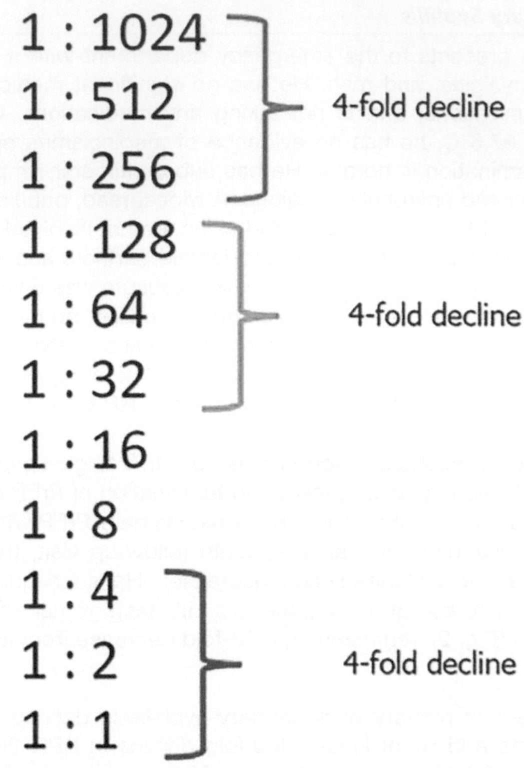

Fig. 3. RPR titer dilutions and examples of fourfold (two dilutions) decreases in titer values.

Providing patients with documentation (such as in **Table 2**) of their syphilis stage, serologic results, and treatment history can empower patients and reduce the likelihood of unnecessary treatment when they undergo future testing.

Vignette 3: Late Latent Syphilis

A 27-year-old man presents to his primary care provider for follow-up STI screening. The patient has a history of syphilis of unknown duration, diagnosed 24 months ago, which was his first visit for STI screening in 3 years. Twenty-four months ago, he reported no genital ulcers, rashes, or other characteristic syphilis symptoms. His physical examination was unremarkable, with no urogenital or mucosal ulcers, rash, or

Table 2
Sample documentation to provide to a patient with their staging, testing, and treatment history

Date	Syphilis Stage	Serologic Results	Treatment Given	Comments
01/01/2022	Secondary	TP-EIA + RPR 1:128	BPG 2.4 MIU × 1	Diagnosed/treated in Baltimore, MD
04/01/2022	-	RPR 1:64	-	-
01/01/2023	-	RPR 1:4	-	Fully treated with adequate serologic response

neurologic abnormalities. TP-EIA was reactive, an RPR was 1:4, and an HIV antigen/antibody test was nonreactive. He was treated with BPG 7.2 MIU administered as three doses of 2.4 MIU intramuscularly each at 1-week intervals. His two partners were diagnosed with late latent syphilis and treated appropriately, and all abstained from sex for 1 week following treatment. The patient's RPR testing was repeated 6, 12, and 18 months ago and all resulted with a titer of 1:2. Today, he reports no new partners, no genital, dermatologic, neurologic, ocular, or otic symptoms, and the physical examination (including neurologic examination) is unremarkable. An RPR is repeated and is 1:2, and repeat HIV antigen/antibody testing is nonreactive.

Discussion

This patient was treated for syphilis of unknown duration 24 months ago but his follow-up NTT has not undergone a fourfold decline. An appropriate serologic response may not occur after treatment, even in the absence of reinfection.[3] This is termed "inadequate serologic response" and best describes the scenario for the patient above. It is estimated that inadequate serologic response is observed at 12 months in approximately 9.4% of cases of primary and secondary syphilis and in 21% of cases of late latent syphilis.[11] Serologic response has been associated with earlier syphilis stage, whereas lower baseline non-treponemal titers,[12,13] older age,[14] female sex,[15] HIV infection,[16] and previous syphilis infection are associated with longer time to achieve a serologic response.

Inadequate serologic response may be distressing for patients and perplexing for their clinicians. For patients identified with inadequate serologic response, the 2021 CDC treatment guidelines recommend careful clinical assessments (including neurologic examinations) and serologic follow-up annually. CSF examination may be considered where follow-up is uncertain or initial high titers (>1:32) do not decrease after 24 months, to determine if asymptomatic neurosyphilis may be the reason for serologic nonresponse. There is currently no evidence for improved clinical outcomes to support additional treatment for patients with inadequate serologic response in the absence of neurosyphilis.[10] However, if ongoing follow-up cannot be assured or if the initial titer was high (>1:32) and does not decrease at least fourfold, it is recommended to retreat with 3 weekly injections of 2.4 MIU of BPG.[3]

It is important to differentiate "inadequate serologic response" from "treatment failure." Concern for treatment failure occurs when there is at least a fourfold *sustained* increase in NTT titer persisting for greater than 2 weeks without signs or symptoms attributable to primary or secondary syphilis, when reinfection is considered unlikely. Along with reevaluation for HIV infection, for patients with treatment failure who have neurologic findings, or who have no neurologic findings and no sexual exposure during the previous year, a CSF examination is recommended.[3] Treatment depends on CSF findings. Among persons with no neurologic findings after neurologic examination and who are sexually active, treatment with weekly injections of BPG 2.4 MIU IM for 3 weeks is recommended.

In this case, as the patient is able to attend follow-up visits, it would be appropriate to continue follow-up serology and clinical examination annually or more frequently based on changes in sexual exposures, to evaluate for new syphilis symptoms.

Vignette 4: Neurosyphilis

A 68-year-old woman with a past medical history of well-controlled hypertension and a transient ischemic attack 10 years earlier presents to clinic with her family. She has a 3-year history of increasing forgetfulness with personality change and now regularly misplaces objects at home and has subsequently stopped driving. She endorses intermittent, stabbing bilateral lower extremity pains associated with numbness. She endorses vision changes which had been previously attributed to cataracts. On physical examination, she has right-sided anisocoria and reduced sensation to pinprick and light touch in her bilateral lower extremities with diminished reflexes. Eye examination is limited by bilateral cataracts; a formal ophthalmologic examination reveals no additional findings.

She is found to have a reactive TT with an RPR titer of 1:2. She cannot recall prior treatment for syphilis and the local health department does not have a record of prior syphilis treatment. She reports no sexual encounters within the past year.

After a shared decision-making conversation with the patient and her family, an examination of her cerebrospinal fluid (CSF) is obtained and is notable for lymphocytic pleocytosis (36 white blood cells per microliter) and a CSF total protein of 56 mg/dL; CSF-VDRL is nonreactive. She was treated with aqueous crystalline penicillin 24 MIU intravenously per day for a total of 14 days. On day 14, she received a subsequent dose of 2.4 MIU of intramuscular BPG. At 12 and 24 months follow-up, the RPR was nonreactive. Her forgetfulness had not worsened; the pain in her legs had resolved and there were no new visual complaints. A repeat CSF examination was not obtained per guidelines.

Discussion

This patient had late neurosyphilis as manifested by general paresis and tabes dorsalis. Neurologic syphilis encompasses a vast spectrum of clinical manifestations and importantly can occur at any point during infection with TP. Patients with early neurosyphilis (typically within 1 year of infection) are more likely to present with meningitis, stroke, and cranial nerve palsies. Late neurosyphilis (initial infection occurred greater than 1 year ago or is unknown) is a tertiary manifestation of infection and classically includes the progressive dementia known as general paresis as well as posterior spinal column disease, termed tabes dorsalis. Of note, ocular and otic syphilis can occur at any stage of syphilis infection, in conjunction with neurosyphilis or in isolation, and are often considered distinct entities.

The diagnosis of neurosyphilis is challenging; there is no single test with robust enough characteristics alone to confirm or refute the diagnosis in all scenarios. CSF findings include lymphocytic pleocytosis, an elevated CSF protein, and a reactive CSF-VDRL. The CSF-VDRL lacks sensitivity (estimated to be 49%–87.5%) and can be negative in those who otherwise are considered to have neurosyphilis.[6] In individuals with a negative CSF-VDRL and suspected neurosyphilis, CSF FTA-ABS may be conducted. The CSF FTA-ABS is up to 100% sensitive but less specific than CSF-VDRL.[17,18] Some experts believe that a negative CSF-FTA-ABS excludes neurosyphilis, particularly in a person with nonspecific neurologic symptoms.

Primary care providers are routinely the first to identify and attempt to establish an etiology for cognitive decline in our communities. It is therefore important to note that syphilis serologies are not universally recommended as a means of screening for all patients in this setting.[19] Instead, we recommend that exposure history, epidemiologic factors, and associated neurologic signs and symptoms are considered before the initiation of testing.

Regardless, the primary care provider may be tasked with determining if CSF examination for an elderly patient with reactive serologies is truly necessary. Patients with neurologic signs and symptoms (ie, cranial nerve deficits, meningitis, stroke, altered mental status, cognitive decline, loss of vibration sense, or proprioception) in the context of reactive syphilis serologies should undergo CSF testing. As outlined in our case, we recommend that a shared decision-making model is used when considering a CSF examination for an elderly patient, taking into account both the procedure and the potential treatment.

In patients with isolated ocular or otic symptoms who have no evidence of neurosyphilis (ie, headache, altered mental status, cranial nerve deficit), CSF testing can be avoided. Instead, focused ophthalmologic or otologic evaluation should be pursued. As many as 30% of patients with ocular syphilis and 90% with otic syphilis have normal CSF.[20,21]

Vignette 5: Syphilis in Pregnancy

A 28-year-old primigravida presents for routine prenatal care at 30 weeks gestation. She recently moved and is attending a new clinic in a different state. She has no significant medical history, no history of syphilis, and prenatal fetal anomaly scans were normal. She has had one male sexual partner for the past 4 years. HIV, RPR via traditional testing algorithm, chlamydia, and gonorrhea were nonreactive or negative at her first prenatal visit.

Her laboratory results from this visit reveal a reactive TT by the reverse sequence algorithm, which is the standard of care in her new jurisdiction. Reflex RPR was nonreactive and a second, different TT was also reactive. On further evaluation, she has no signs or symptoms of syphilis and the physical examination is normal. Her partner tested negative for syphilis. With her testing results, she is diagnosed with syphilis of unknown duration and treated (starting at 31-week gestation) with 2.4 MIU of BPG on days 0, 7, and 14. A repeat fetal ultrasound is normal. She delivers a healthy female neonate at 40 weeks. Maternal RPR remains negative at delivery. The neonate has a normal physical examination and nonreactive serum RPR.

Discussion

Syphilis diagnosed in pregnancy must prompt additional evaluation of the fetus for CS. The diagnosis of CS is based on a combination of factors: maternal syphilis serology interpretation, adequacy of maternal treatment and timing before delivery, presence of clinical, laboratory, or radiographic evidence of syphilis in the neonate, and comparison of maternal (at delivery) and neonatal NTT titers. These factors guide classification of CS and management.[3] CS is more likely to occur if the pregnant person has primary or secondary syphilis. However, it can occur at any stage of syphilis in the pregnant person, including during latent infection. CS is preventable by providing adequate access to screening and treatment during pregnancy. Parenteral penicillin is the only acceptable treatment in pregnancy. Pregnant people who are allergic to penicillin should be desensitized and receive stage-appropriate treatment.

This case demonstrates the challenges associated with using an alternate syphilis diagnostic algorithm during prenatal care. If the patient had ongoing prenatal care in her previous jurisdiction and continued to be tested with the RPR, a diagnosis of syphilis in pregnancy would have been missed. It has been observed that screening with the reverse algorithm identifies additional true positives and false positives, though the proportions vary by population disease prevalence.[9]

Fortunately, this patient was diagnosed at 30 weeks and completed stage-appropriate treatment by week 34. Her neonate was born more than 30 days after she completed therapy, thereby avoiding an automatic diagnosis of CS.[3] A more challenging scenario is when a pregnant person, with a nonreactive RPR, is tested for the first time using the reverse algorithm late in the third trimester or at delivery; there is insufficient opportunity to complete stage-appropriate treatment before delivery. States have implemented varied recommendations for the frequency of screening for syphilis during pregnancy; clinicians should be familiar with the requirements in their jurisdiction.[22]

Vignette 6: Biologic False Positive

A 50-year-old woman attends a routine gynecology appointment for preventive care. She has never been diagnosed with an STI and has not been sexually active since her last testing 5 years ago, when her syphilis screening (via reverse algorithm) was nonreactive. She undergoes Pap testing that is normal and STI screening, which includes syphilis testing by the traditional sequence algorithm. The RPR is reactive, with a titer of 1:4, and a TP-PA is nonreactive. Tests for *N gonorrhea, C trachomatis*, and HIV are nonreactive. She is referred for mammography, is identified with a breast mass and is diagnosed with locally advanced breast cancer. Her primary care provider conducts a careful examination which is normal, reviews the patient's sexual history, RPR and TP-PA results, and determines that no syphilis treatment is needed.

Discussion

This patient has discrepant NTT and TT results performed by the traditional algorithm. In the absence of signs/symptoms suggestive of syphilis, or recent exposure, this patient's combination of results in the traditional algorithm is consistent with a "biologic false positive (BFP)." See **Table 3**, for a summary of possible interpretations of TT and NTT combinations.

BFP results are observed among NTT and TT. The prevalence of BFP results depends on the population tested but has been reported to account for 11% to 40% of reactive NTTs in surveillance data (including people with indications for screening)[23] and at much lower rates in the general population (<1%).[24]

A variety of epidemiologic factors and clinical conditions has been associated with BFPs, though the presence of BFP does not require association with any condition and does not portend an occult condition; in the absence of suggestive symptoms or epidemiologic exposures, no additional workup is required. BFP NTT has been associated with older age, female sex, autoimmune conditions (classically systemic lupus erythematosus), hematologic conditions, malignancy, HIV, and hepatitis C.[23–26] Infections (including Lyme disease), autoimmune conditions, and older age have been associated with BFP TT.[10] BFP association with pregnancy is controversial and every effort should be made to exclude syphilis in a pregnant person; expert consultation is recommended.

Attribution of reactive NTT or TT as a BFP should occur when other clues to a potential syphilis infection have been assessed and excluded. In this case, the patient has no

Table 3
Summary of treponemal test and non-treponemal test results and possible interpretations

Non-treponemal RPR (or VDRL)	Treponemal (FTA, TP-PA, and EIA)	Possible Interpretation
Reactive	Nonreactive	Biologic false-positive NTT False-negative TT
Reactive	Reactive	New diagnosis—requires treatment Old case – adequately treated Old case—inadequately treated Previously treated—reinfected Congenital Other treponematoses (eg, Yaws)
Nonreactive	Reactive	Primary syphilis before NTT are positive Old case—treated or untreated Prozone reaction (uncommon)
Nonreactive	Nonreactive	No syphilis Incubating syphilis/seronegative primary syphilis

recent sexual exposure, no clinical signs of syphilis, and a potential underlying condition (malignancy) that could be related to the BFP. In situations where the concern for syphilis is elevated based on epidemiologic factors, exposure, or examination findings, some experts may complete a second, different TT, following the reactive RPR and nonreactive TT completed in the traditional algorithm. If the second TT is reactive, the patient should be assessed and treated for syphilis consistent with the clinical stage.

SUMMARY

This series of vignettes highlights the concepts in syphilis serologic interpretation. Even with this guidance, the interpretation of syphilis serologies is complex and can be ambiguous; definitive criteria for cure or failure by serologic assessment have not been well established.[3] Several resources are available to assist clinicians in syphilis management. The 2021 CDC Sexually Transmitted Infection (STI) Treatment guidelines outline screening, interpretation, and treatment recommendations.[3] The National STD Curriculum (std.uw.edu) is a free educational Web site with self-study lessons and a question bank. The CDC National Network of STI Clinical Prevention Training Centers (NNPTCs) offer a free STI Clinical Consultation Service (stdccn.org) that provides expert advice over email or telephone on specific patient scenarios. For health care professionals in the United States, the NNPTCs offer training on STI prevention topics (https://www.cdc.gov/std/projects/nnptc.htm). Local health departments play a vital role in maintaining testing and treatment histories for reportable conditions, including syphilis. Clinicians should familiarize themselves with their local health department contacts to retrieve records and get assistance with requests from other jurisdictions. Finally, infectious diseases clinicians will have experience in the interpretation of syphilis serology and should be consulted for advice when appropriate.

CLINICS CARE POINTS

- Interpretation of syphilis serology can be challenging even for experienced providers.
- Diagnosis of syphilis relies on reactive treponemal-specific and non-treponemal antibody testing and clinical assessment.
- Serologic antibody testing may be nonreactive early in infection, leading to false-negative results.
- Ensure adequate time has passed (12 months for primary and secondary syphilis, 24 months for latent syphilis) before making a decision about serologic treatment success.
- Lumbar puncture is only indicated in specific scenarios, such as when a patient has neurologic symptoms or non-treponemal test titers increase ≥4-fold in the absence of reexposure.
- Local health departments can often provide a syphilis testing and treatment history
- Remember to test for HIV and offer HIV pre-exposure prophylaxis to patients with syphilis.

DISCLOSURE

The authors have no financial disclosures or conflicts of interest to disclose.

REFERENCES

1. Centers for Disease Control and Prevention (CDC). Sexually Transmitted Disease Surveillance 2021. Atlanta: US Department of Health and Human Services; 2023.

2. Seña AC, White BL, Sparling PF. Novel *Treponema pallidum* serologic tests: a paradigm shift in syphilis screening for the 21st century. Clin Infect Dis 2010; 51(6):700–8.
3. Workowski K, Bachmann L, Chan P, et al. Sexually Transmitted Infections Treatment Guidelines, 2021. MMWR Recomm Rep (Morb Mortal Wkly Rep) 2021; 70(4):1–187.
4. Henao-Martínez AF, Johnson SC. Diagnostic tests for syphilis: New tests and new algorithms. Neurol Clin Pract 2014;4(2):114.
5. Romanowski B, Sutherland R, Fick GH, et al. Serologic response to treatment of infectious syphilis. Ann Intern Med 1991;114(12):1005–9.
6. Tuddenham S, Katz SS, Ghanem KG. Syphilis Laboratory Guidelines: Performance Characteristics of Nontreponemal Antibody Tests. Clin Infect Dis 2020; 71(Suppl 1):S21–42.
7. Sparling PF, Swartz M, Musher D, et al. Clinical manifestations of syphilis. In: Holmes KK, Sparling PF, Stamm WE, et al, editors. Sexually transmitted diseases. 4th edition. New York: McGrawHill; 2008. p. 661–84.
8. Towns JM, Leslie DE, Denham I, et al. Painful and multiple anogenital lesions are common in men with *Treponema pallidum* PCR-positive primary syphilis without herpes simplex virus coinfection: a cross-sectional clinic-based study. Sex Transm Infect 2016;92(2):110–5.
9. Cantor AG, Pappas M, Daeges M, et al. Screening for Syphilis: Updated Evidence Report and Systematic Review for the US Preventive Services Task Force. JAMA 2016;315(21):2328–37.
10. Ghanem KG, Ram S, Rice PA. The Modern Epidemic of Syphilis. N Engl J Med 2020;382(9):845–54.
11. Seña AC, Zhang XH, Li T, et al. A systematic review of syphilis serological treatment outcomes in HIV-infected and HIV-uninfected persons: rethinking the significance of serological non-responsiveness and the serofast state after therapy. BMC Infect Dis 2015;15(1).
12. Li J, Wang LN, Zheng HY. Predictors of serological cure and serofast state after treatment in HIV-negative patients with early syphilis in China. Sex Transm Infect 2013;89(1):69.
13. Jinno S, Anker B, Kaur P, et al. Predictors of serological failure after treatment in HIV-infected patients with early syphilis in the emerging era of universal antiretroviral therapy use. BMC Infect Dis 2013;13(1).
14. QIN J, YANG T, WANG H, et al. Potential Predictors for Serofast State after Treatment among HIV-Negative Persons with Syphilis in China: A Systematic Review and Meta-Analysis. Iran J Public Health 2015;44(2):155.
15. Tong ML, Lin LR, Liu GL, et al. Factors associated with serological cure and the serofast state of HIV-negative patients with primary, secondary, latent, and tertiary syphilis. PLoS One 2013;8(7).
16. Luo Z, Zhu L, Ding Y, et al. Factors associated with syphilis treatment failure and reinfection: a longitudinal cohort study in Shenzhen, China. BMC Infect Dis 2017;17(1).
17. Jaffe HW, Larsen SA, Peters M, et al. Tests for Treponemal Antibody in CSF. Arch Intern Med 1978;138(2):252–5.
18. Park IU, Tran A, Pereira L, et al. Sensitivity and Specificity of Treponemal-specific Tests for the Diagnosis of Syphilis. Clin Infect Dis 2020;71(Suppl 1):S13–20.
19. Knopman DS, DeKosky ST, Cummings JL, et al. Practice parameter: diagnosis of dementia (an evidence-based review). Report of the Quality Standards Subcommittee of the American Academy of Neurology. Neurology 2001;56(9):1143–53.

20. Yimtae K, Srirompotong S, Lertsukprasert K. Otosyphilis: a review of 85 cases. Otolaryngol Head Neck Surg 2007;136(1):67–71.
21. Lapere S, Mustak H, Steffen J. Clinical Manifestations and Cerebrospinal Fluid Status in Ocular Syphilis. Ocul Immunol Inflamm 2019;27(1):126–30.
22. CDC. Division of STD Prevention (DSTDP) State Statutory and Regulatory Language Regarding Prenatal Syphilis Screenings in the United States. Available at: https://www.cdc.gov/std/treatment/syphilis-screenings.htm. Published 2020. Accessed June 18, 2023.
23. Matthias J, Klingler EJ, Schillinger JA, et al. Frequency and Characteristics of Biological False-Positive Test Results for Syphilis Reported in Florida and New York City, USA, 2013 to 2017. J Clin Microbiol 2019;57(11).
24. Liu F, Liu LL, Guo XJ, et al. Characterization of the classical biological false-positive reaction in the serological test for syphilis in the modern era. Int Immunopharmacol 2014;20(2):331–6.
25. Augenbraun M, French A, Glesby M, et al. Hepatitis C virus infection and biological false-positive syphilis tests. Sex Transm Infect 2010;86(2):97–8.
26. Rompalo AM, Cannon RO, Quinn TC, et al. Association of biologic false-positive reactions for syphilis with human immunodeficiency virus infection. J Infect Dis 1992;165(6):1124–6.

Proctitis

An Approach to the Symptomatic Patient

Candice J. McNeil, MD, MPH[a,*], Luis F. Barroso II, MD[a],
Kimberly Workowski, MD[b]

KEYWORDS

• Proctitis • Sexually transmitted infection • Treatment • Prevention

KEY POINTS

- Proctitis is an inflammatory condition of the distal rectum.
- Common sexually transmitted infections, such as gonorrhea, chlamydia, and syphilis, may be associated with proctitis.
- Data are evolving around the role of *Mycoplasma genitalium* and other pathogens in proctitis.
- New pathogens, such as Mpox, should be considered in select clinical scenarios.
- The Centers for Disease Control and Prevention Guidelines are a resource for providers to facilitate the diagnosis, treatment, and prevention of sexually transmitted infections and associated clinical syndromes such as proctitis.

DISEASE MANIFESTATIONS AND EPIDEMIOLOGY

Proctitis is an inflammatory disease of the distal rectum that includes the hallmark findings of rectal discharge, anorectal pain, and tenesmus (the reoccurring urge to have a bowel movement). Anal sexual exposures, including genital, digital, and/or oral-anal contact, are associated with the clinical syndrome of proctitis.[1] Most of the published literature on proctitis focuses on populations of men who have sex with men (MSM), or other gay or bisexual men. The differential diagnosis of proctitis includes noninfectious causes, such as inflammatory bowel disease, radiation or chemical proctitis, and ischemia. Sexually transmitted causes of proctitis include *Neisseria gonorrhoeae* (NG), *Chlamydia trachomatis* (CT; Lymphogranuloma venereum [LGV] and non-Lymphogranuloma venereum serovars), *Mycoplasma genitalium* (MG), and *Treponema pallidum* (the pathogen associated with syphilis).[1] When

[a] Department of Medicine, Section on Infectious Diseases, Wake Forest University School of Medicine; [b] Department of Medicine, Division of Infectious Diseases, Emory University School of Medicine
* Corresponding author. Wake Forest University School of Medicine, Medical Center Boulevard, Winston Salem, NC 27157.
E-mail address: cmcneil@wakehealth.edu

Med Clin N Am 108 (2024) 339–354
https://doi.org/10.1016/j.mcna.2023.09.002 medical.theclinics.com

bloody discharge, perianal, and mucosal ulcerations are present, in addition to LGV and herpes simplex virus (HSV), Mpox (formerly monkeypox) is in the differential.[1] Other bacterial and viral pathogens also can cause proctitis, and multiple pathogens can also occur concurrently.

Common Sexually Transmitted Bacterial Infections Associated with Proctitis

Notably, studies describing the composition of bacterial pathogens associated with proctitis in the United States have highlighted a stable distribution of bacterial sexually transmitted infections (STIs), such as NG (20%–24%), CT (11%–23%), and syphilis (1%–4%),[2,3] suggesting that these pathogens should continue to be prioritized in terms of diagnostics and empiric treatment.

Rectal CT and NG are common infections in STI care settings. Most asymptomatic CT infection in these instances are caused by serovars D-K, non-LGV forms of chlamydia. It is not uncommon for these infections to occur at the rectal site particularly in MSM who engage in receptive anal sex. Although they can cause symptomatic proctitis, most of these infections are asymptomatic. Asymptomatic CT and NG rectal infections are known to occur in women where reported anal receptive intercourse is not a prerequisite.[4–6] The proximity of the vagina to the anus is a factor contributing to autoinoculation, with the rectal site continuing to serve a reservoir if not appropriately treated.[4] Although it is feasible that an asymptomatic infection at the rectum in a woman may progress to symptomatic proctitis, most data on this clinical syndrome have been described among MSM. When proctitis occurs, it is not possible to clinically distinguish NG from CT based on examination findings, although LGV serovars L1–L3 of chlamydia are more common when symptomatic rectal CT infections are identified.[1]

The clinical findings of LGV associated with anorectal disease include transient ulcer formation, inguinal lymphadenopathy, hemorrhagic rectal discharge, often presenting as the clinical syndrome of proctocolitis. Those with proctocolitis may have symptoms of proctitis plus gastrointestinal symptoms, such as abdominal cramps, diarrhea, and colonic inflammation.[1,7] In addition to LGV, the differential diagnosis of STIs causing proctocolitis includes enteric pathogens, such as *Campylobacter* species, *Shigella* species, *Entamoeba histolytica*, and in immunocompromised persons, cytomegalovirus (CMV).[1,8] Inadequately treated LGV infections can lead to complications including invasive disease with potential for chronic colorectal complaints, such as fistula, and fissure can occur.[1,7] The true prevalence of LGV infection in the United States is unknown owing to the reliance on clinical diagnosis, as LGV diagnostics are not readily available and serologic tests are unreliable. Providers should therefore assume the diagnosis of LGV when there is a positive rectal nucleic acid amplification test (NAAT) for CT in a person with symptoms, epidemiologic findings, and clinical features consistent with LGV, and other potential causes of proctocolitis have been ruled out.[1] Concomitant infection with HIV is known to occur.[9,10] In a cluster of LGV cases in Michigan, 16% of the 38 cases had incident HIV. Concurrent STIs, including gonorrhea and syphilis, were identified along with hepatitis C. Half of the cases had the clinical presentation of proctitis.[9] A recent retrospective review of MSM with CT in New York found LGV was found to be significantly associated with age greater than or equal to 30, non-Hispanic black race, history of syphilis, having a partner with HIV, and living with HIV.[10] Anorectal symptoms were common in this study with 63% (n = 186) of persons whose anorectal CT specimens were tested noted to be symptomatic at the time of specimen collection.[10] Twenty-three percent of these symptomatic persons had LGV. Among the signs or symptoms reviewed, rectal discharge had the highest sensitivity and was associated with the highest positive predictive value for an LGV diagnosis.[10]

Syphilis can manifest various clinical presentations and[11,12] poses a unique diagnostic challenge to even a seasoned clinician. Syphilis infection of the lower gastrointestinal tract may mimic several conditions, leading to delayed or missed diagnosis.[12,13] Ferzacca and colleagues[13] described 62 cases of lower gastrointestinal tract syphilis in men and transgender women for which HIV was a common comorbidity in 26 cases. Nontreponemal serology titers for cases ranged from 1:2 to 1:1024. The most common presenting symptom was hematochezia (67%). Other anorectal symptoms included anal pain (46%), tenesmus (25%), and mucus discharge (23%). Other findings included abdominal pain (28%), diarrhea (23%), constipation (13%), weight loss (10%), fever (8%), and anal ulceration (7%). In addition, rash, myalgia, arthralgia, anal mass, anorexia, headache, and pruritus were reported.[13] Physical examination findings included rectal mass (38%), lymphadenopathy (31%), rash (26%), unknown (14%), and perianal ulceration (7%). There were other local anorectal findings (lesions, tenderness) in 5% or less of subjects.[13] The variability of findings lends to the challenges of syphilis diagnosis at the anorectal site and reinforced the importance of completing a comprehensive sexual history to assess for potential exposures, using the appropriate serologic and supportive diagnostics, direct visualization, and biopsy with histopathology as needed for diagnosis. The concurrency of HIV in this cohort also reinforces the need for comprehensive STI/HIV testing.

The Role of Other Bacterial Pathogens

Although rare, *Neisseria meningitidis* (NM) has been associated with sexual transmission owing to nongroupable strains and some invasive strains in men who have sex with women. It has also been associated with rectal colonization and symptomatic anorectal disease in women and MSM, although more commonly the latter. Coinfection with NG has also been reported in outbreaks and sporadic infections of NM along with other STIs, including HIV.[14] Notably, NM can colonize the oral pharynx; in the case of urogenital and anogenital infection, it is proposed to be transmitted via oral sex in heterosexuals and MSM.[15]

MG, a pathogen with a known association with symptomatic urogenital disease, has been identified in rectal specimens of persons presenting for STI-related complaints. The understanding of the contribution of MG to symptomatic anorectal disease is evolving. Read and colleagues[16] found that MG, although more common at the rectum compared with the urethra in MSM presenting for sexual health services, was not associated with proctitis in their studied population. Similarly, Soni and colleagues[17] in a population of MSM presenting for screening did not see an association with anorectal symptoms and MG infection. Francis and colleagues in a pilot cross-section study in San Francisco did however note an association between coinfection with CT, rectal symptoms, and proctitis with MG. However, in the multivariate analysis, HIV infection was strongly associated with MG.[18] A more recent study by Chow and colleagues[19] identified MG as a pathogen contributing to proctitis. Furthermore, MG was reported by Ong and colleagues[20] to be nearly as common as CT (17% vs 21%, respectively) infection and less common than NG (40%), and coinfection with other STIs was 22%. The clinical manifestations of MG had less pain than CT and NG. Interestingly, persons with MG coinfection were more likely to report pain than persons with MG monoinfection. However, a portion of those with complaints of pain with coinfection had HSV infection (38%).[20] In this same study, MG infection had significantly higher numbers of persons with HIV than persons with CT or NG monoinfection.[20] MG is not a reportable disease in the United States, and the true prevalence is unknown. Surveillance studies are underway to better understand clinical presentation of MG among men and women presenting for STI care in the United States. Testing for MG is recommended in instances of persistent or recurrent proctitis when standard treatment regimens have failed.[1] Additional details on MG are available in the article in this issue by ("Mycoplasma genitalium: Key Information for the Primary Care Clinician").

Several enteric pathogens have been reported to be associated with symptomatic proctitis.[1] *Shigella* spp, associated with the syndrome proctocolitis, has known associations with sexual transmission, concurrent coinfection with common bacterial STIs, and HIV coinfection.[8] A recent study by Chow and colleagues,[19] in a cohort of men presenting with anorectal symptoms, found *Shigella* spp to be more common in symptomatic men than asymptomatic men. These infections did not have diarrhea as a component of their presentation.[19] More data are needed to understand the prevalence of proctitis because of isolated *Shigella* spp in the United States.

Viral Infections

HIV infection has been noted to have an association with several pathogens associated with proctitis.[21] HIV (with the ability of the virus to modulate immune function) can also be associated with more severe manifestations of proctitis in STIs.

HSV is a cause of proctitis. Notably, proctitis associated with HSV can be severe in persons with advanced HIV with the potential complication of recalcitrant or resistant infections.[1] Reliance on the presence of a perianal ulcer may lead to underdiagnoses of proctitis owing to HSV, which may present with intra-anal ulcerations.[3,22] These lesions may be extensive and prone to poor healing. Atypical presentations mimicking neoplasia may occur warranting biopsy to aid in diagnosis. Persons with poor immunologic control of HIV, such as those with CD4 counts less than 100, have the additional potential complication of acyclovir-resistant HSV, supporting the use of culture with resistance testing in persons who fail to respond to standard therapy.[22]

Proctitis associated with Mpox (formerly monkeypox) is a frequent manifestation in the current outbreak in MSM and may be the main or isolated syndrome identified.[23] Anorectal manifestations, including anal and perianal lesions and/or classic lesions associated with Mpox, may be visible in the anal mucosa.[23,24] Atypical presentations have also been reported.[25] Yakubovsky and colleagues,[26] in their cohort of 70 MSM with Mpox, noted more than a third of these men had proctitis. There was a lack of a typical rash in some and an absence of rash in others.[26] Proctitis may be a more common disease presentation in persons with HIV compared with those without.[27] Those with HIV and a past history of syphilis may also be higher risk for proctitis owing to Mpox.[27] Furthermore, the concurrency of other STIs has also been observed.[28] Severe manifestations of Mpox warranting hospitalization have been reported to be more common in persons with advanced HIV.[29,30] Although vaccination has been reported to have some impact on trends, recent data have highlighted outbreaks in vaccinated populations, reminding us of the need to be vigilant of Mpox in the community.[31,32]

INITIAL EVALUATION AND DIAGNOSIS

Safe, effective, patient-centered, timely, efficient, and equitable STI care services are of the utmost importance. To achieve this end, recommendations for providing quality STI services are available to support practitioners in the private and public sector.[33] In patients coming in with complaints concerning for proctitis (eg, discharge, anorectal pain, and tenesmus), the history and physical examinations, together with appropriate laboratory testing, are the mainstay for evaluation (**Table 1** provides initial testing and empiric treatment recommendations).

Table 1
Initial testing and empiric treatment recommendations for proctitis

	Diagnostics	Treatment
Empiric coverage, bacterial STIs, persons *without* bloody anal discharge, perianal, or mucosal ulcerations	Rectal NAAT CT/NG HIV ab/Ag RPR	Ceftriaxone 500 mg IM in persons <150 kg and 1 g IM in persons ≥150 kg AND Doxycycline 100 mg PO bid × 7 d
Empiric coverage, bacterial STIs *with* bloody anal discharge, perianal, or mucosal ulcerations	Rectal NAAT CT/NG HIV ab/Ag RPR HSV PCR lesions Mpox PCR[a] lesion Mpox PCR[a] rectal	Ceftriaxone 500 mg IM in persons <150 kg and 1 g IM in persons ≥150 kg AND Doxycycline 100 mg PO bid × 21 d AND Antiviral coverage anogenital HSV First clinical episode Acyclovir 400 mg orally tid for 7–10 d OR Famciclovir 250 mg orally tid for 7–10 d OR Valacyclovir 1 g orally bid for 7–10 d Episodic therapy for recurrent HSV-2 Acyclovir 800 mg orally bid for 5 d OR Acyclovir 800 mg orally tid for 2 d OR Famciclovir 1 g orally bid for 1 d OR Famciclovir 500 mg once, followed by 250 mg bid for 2 d OR Famciclovir 125 mg bid for 5 d OR Valacyclovir 500 mg orally bid for 3 d OR Valacyclovir 1 g orally once daily for 5 d

Abbreviations: bid, twice daily; IM, intramuscular; PO, by mouth; RPR, rapid plasma reagin; tid, 3 times daily; VDRL, venereal disease research laboratory.

[a] Consider testing if clinical or epidemiologic factors present to support diagnosis. (See Mclean and colleagues in this issue for a detailed review of Mpox.)

The History

A detailed sexual history, past medical history, and patient demographics can assist in the differential diagnosis. For example, STIs are more common among younger male patients, particularly the MSM population[34]; ischemic colitis occurs typically in older patients with vascular disease risk factors, and inflammatory bowel disease has a bimodal age distribution.[35]

The Examination

The physical examination evaluation of proctitis includes inspection of the perianal area for purulence, inflammation, perianal ulcers, and palpation of the anal canal through a thorough a digital anorectal examination. Care should be taken as the examination may be painful in symptomatic patients. Standard anoscopy allows for the identification of the typical signs of proctitis, such as inflamed mucosa and purulence (**Fig. 1**), anal fissure, solitary rectal ulcer, hemorrhoids, or condyloma.[36] Proctosigmoidoscopy allows for more detailed examination of the mucosa and, when appropriate, biopsy of involved tissue may be needed. Practitioners should have access to standard anoscopy and performance of the digital anorectal examination in the evaluation of persons with proctitis. (See the next section for additional details on high-resolution anoscopy.)

Initial Laboratory Evaluation

Examination of anal discharge or exudate collected at the time of anoscopy with a gram-stained smear may be useful to detect the presence of polymorphonuclear cells supporting the diagnosis of proctitis.[1] The laboratory evaluation includes evaluation of bacterial STIs with NAAT testing for gonorrhea and chlamydia, and HSV polymerase chain reaction (PCR) testing of ulcerative lesions if present. Other pathogens can be evaluated with stool culture or molecular testing depending on epidemiologic risk and clinical factors, including Mpox NAAT testing, which can be sent for select patients.

Empiric Treatment

Empiric guideline-based treatment should not be delayed while awaiting laboratory results (see **Table 1** and "Treatment" in later discussion).

HIGH-RESOLUTION ANOSCOPY FINDINGS

High-resolution anoscopy (HRA) involves close inspection of the anal mucosa through a colposcope for the diagnosis and treatment of high-grade squamous intraepithelial (HSIL) lesions of the anus. Treatment of anal HSIL has been shown to decrease incidence of anal squamous cell carcinoma in people living with HIV.[37] During the procedure, 5% acetic acid and iodine (Lugol) solution are applied to highlight lesions. The procedure takes approximately 5 to 20 minutes.[38]

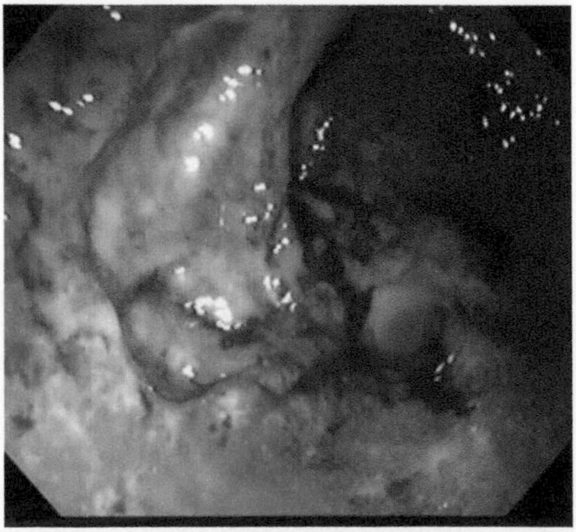

Fig. 1. Anoscopy with purulence and friability consistent with proctitis.

Although HRA is generally well-tolerated as a screening procedure in an asymptomatic population, in the setting of proctitis, the inflammation and pain can make HRA more challenging. As noted, standard anoscopy without magnification, acetic acid, or Lugol, is the recommended diagnostic procedure for the most patients with proctitis.

Despite this, the high-risk cohorts that require HRA for anal dysplasia screening often also have a high incidence of proctitis, so the HRA procedure may be performed serendipitously. HRA findings in proctitis are nonspecific and include friable mucosa, purulent discharge, dilated looped vessels, and pain on examination (**Figs. 2** and **3**). Shallow ulcers may be noted in certain causes, such as HSV proctitis or LGV (see **Fig. 2**; **Figs. 4** and **5**). Vesicles may be seen in Mpox or HSV. Biopsies often show nonspecific inflammation but may reveal specific pathogens, such as HSV or CMV, on immunostaining. Thus, although HRA is not part of the standard evaluation for proctitis, there are important diagnostic clues that can be observed in the HRA examination. HRA practitioners should be familiar with the signs and symptoms of proctitis as well as the HRA findings of appropriate diagnostic testing empiric treatment.

TREATMENT

Empiric treatment of proctitis (see **Table 1**) in sexually active persons is targeted toward the most commonly identified pathogens and includes highly effective regimens for CT and NG.[1,39] Regimens covering NG are likely to be effective against NM. **Table 2** provides diagnostics and treatments suggested for specific pathogens associated with proctitis.

Several studies have now demonstrated a superiority of doxycycline for the treatment of chlamydia infections at the rectal site,[40,41] translating into changes in the current Centers for Disease Control and Prevention (CDC) STI guidelines recommendations. Thus, in instances where doxycycline is not used for treatment of rectal CT infection, a test of cure should be performed in 4 weeks to assess the adequacy of treatment.[1] Considering that the rectum could potentially serve as a reservoir for women, doxycycline is also the preferred treatment for this population regardless of rectal exposure.[1] Shared decision-making models accounting to factors such as adherence, cost, anatomic locations covered, and others may dictate whether single-dose azithromycin versus doxycycline may be used for asymptomatic CT

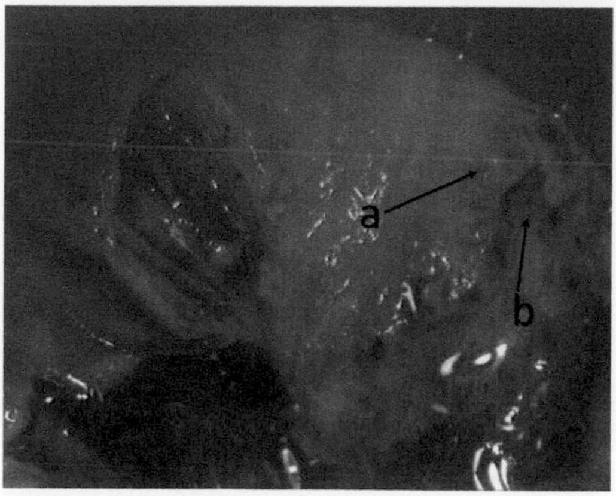

Fig. 2. HRA examination, 5% acetic acid 16×. Thickening of the squamocolumnar junction with purulence, dilated vessels (a), and shallow ulcers (b) are seen.

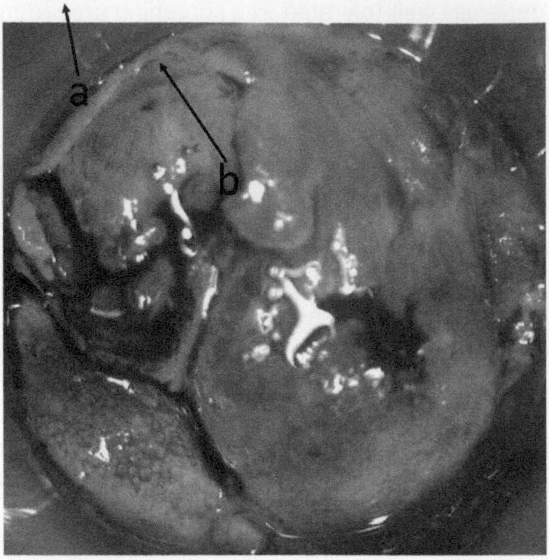

Fig. 3. HRA examination, Lugol solution 16×. Thickened squamocolumnar junction (a) with friable, inflamed mucosa and hypervascularity (b).

infection.[1] Symptomatic rectal infection in the setting of positive rectal CT NAAT and other specific clinical findings may suggest LGV. Given the paucity of diagnostics to confirm this diagnosis, clinical suspicion should prompt providers to treat with a course of doxycycline to encompass the diagnosis of LGV. Although shorter durations of doxycycline have been shown to be effective in limited studies, more data are needed.[42] Thus, the preferred treatment of LGV serovars of CT involves an extended course of doxycycline of 21 days.[43]

Persons presenting with classic symptoms of proctitis with a hemorrhagic component or with the presence of ulcerations should be treated for LGV. Treatment of HSV (which can also cause these symptoms) should be initiated as well. Consideration should be made for the possibility of Mpox. Testing should be performed when feasible to direct and monitor therapy, and in the instance of Mpox, direct control

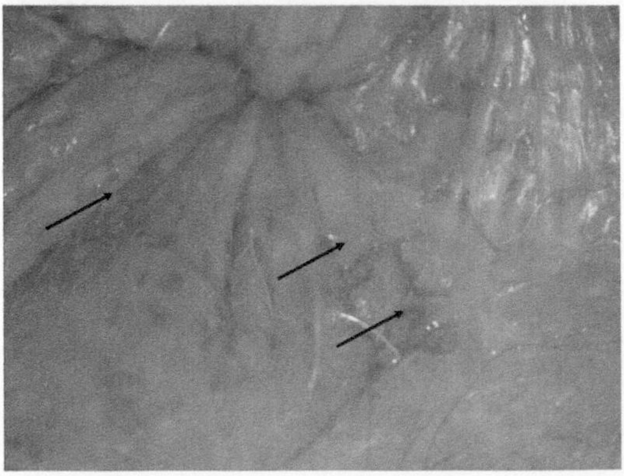

Fig. 4. Perianal HRA examination, 5% acetic acid 10×. Although nondiagnostic, these shallow ulcers were seen in a patient with HSV (*arrows*).

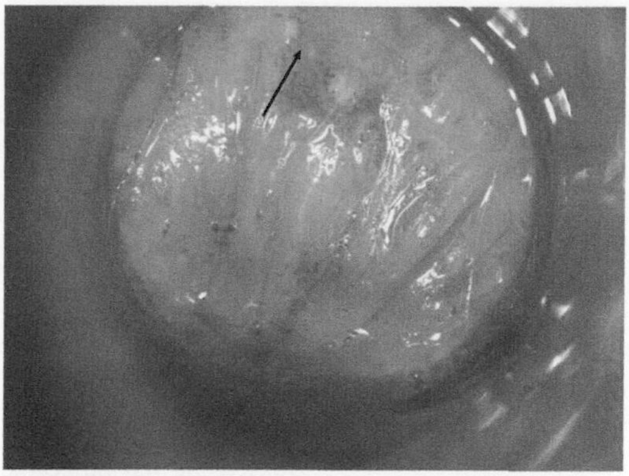

Fig. 5. HRA examination, 5% acetic acid 10×. Shallow serpiginous ulcer seen at the anal verge (*arrow*) in a patient with HSV.

measures and supportive care should be performed when feasible. **Tables 1** and **2** provide primary treatment regimens for HSV and treatment regimens for Mpox. Mclean and colleagues in this issue provide a detailed review of Mpox.

The preferred treatment for syphilis infection is intramuscular benzathine penicillin in the form of a single dose for early syphilis,[1] the stage where symptomatic proctitis may present. Alternative regimes with doxycycline or ceftriaxone can be considered when benzathine penicillin is not available.[44]

MG, a pathogen with a surprisingly high prevalence and alarming trends toward resistance, requires a unique attention to regimen selection.[45,46] Current CDC guidelines recommend that resistance-guided therapy be used; however, this is rarely available in US clinical practice.[1] This leaves treatment with doxycycline to dampen bacterial load followed by moxifloxacin for treatment. However, there are growing trends toward fluoroquinolone resistance, suggesting that other regimes may be needed to affect cure in the future.[1] Notably, because of the fact that both doxycycline and fluoroquinolones are not used in pregnant women in sexual health settings, infectious disease consultation should be sought to design a treatment regimen and follow-up plan should there be a need to treat proctitis in this population. Obefemi and colleagues in this issue provide a detailed review of MG.

PREVENTION

Understanding current risk for STIs via a detailed risk assessment is a leading tool in preventing the recurrence of STIs, including HIV. The 5 P's is a framework by which a provider may be able to ask the right questions to establish the risk baseline of the clients they serve. These questions are outlined succinctly in the 2021 STI guidelines.[1] Providers may consider asking additional questions, which may drive risk behaviors and care decisions, including questions surrounding agency, specifically, an understanding as to whether the client feels safe in their sexual relationships to make the best decisions for their health and well-being. In addition, asking questions about pleasure may identify practices that may be modifiable, including, for instance, the use of lubricant to avoid mucosal tears, the use of lubricants that may increase the risk of STI exposures, such as those that are irritative or those that may convey disease (ie, saliva), and lack of barrier protection use. Augmenting this with other established behavioral counseling techniques may improve the likelihood of success.

Table 2
Proctitis pathogens with associated diagnostics and treatments

Pathogen	Diagnostics	Treatment
C trachomatis (non-LGV)	Rectal NAAT CT	Preferred: doxycycline 100 mg PO bid × 7 d (asymptomatic) Alternative: azithromycin 1 g PO once
LGV	Clinical findings consistent AND Rectal NAAT CT	Preferred: Doxycycline 100 mg PO bid × 21 d Alternative: Azithromycin 1g PO Q week × 3
Ngonorrhoeae[a]	Rectal NAAT NG	Preferred: Ceftriaxone 500 mg IM in persons <150 kg and 1 g IM in persons ≥150 kg AND Doxycycline 100 mg PO bid × 7 d Alternative: *IM cephalosporin not available* Cefixime 800 mg PO once AND Doxycycline 100 mg PO bid × 7 d *IgE-mediated allergy to penicillin or cephalosporin* Gentamicin 240 mg IM × 1 and Azithromycin 2 g PO × 1
T pallidum	[b]Treponemal test (RPR or VDRL) with confirmatory treponemal test OR Nontreponemal test reverse sequence	Preferred: *Primary/secondary/early syphilis*, Benzathine penicillin G 2.4 million units IM × 1 Alternative: Doxycycline 100 mg PO bid × 14 d
Mgenitalium	Rectal NAAT MG	Preferred: *M genitalium* detected by an FDA-cleared NAAT Resistance testing available: • If macrolide resistant: Doxycycline 100 mg orally bid × 7 d, THEN moxifloxacin 400 mg orally once daily × 7 d • If macrolide sensitive: Doxycycline 100 mg orally bid × 7 d, followed by azithromycin 1 g orally initial dose, followed by 500 mg orally once daily for 3 additional days (2.5 g total) Resistance testing not available: Doxycycline 100 mg bid × 7 d, THEN moxifloxacin 400 mg orally once daily × 7 d
Herpes simplex virus	HSV PCR lesion	Antiviral coverage anogenital HSV First clinical episode of herpes Acyclovir 400 mg orally tid × 7–10 d OR Famciclovir 250 mg orally tid × 7–10 d OR Valacyclovir 1 g orally bid × 7–10 d Episodic therapy for recurrent HSV-2 Acyclovir 800 mg orally bid for 5 d

(*continued on next page*)

Table 2
(*continued*)

Pathogen	Diagnostics	Treatment
		OR Acyclovir 800 mg orally tid for 2 d OR Famciclovir 1 g orally bid for 1 d OR Famciclovir 500 mg once, followed by 250 mg 2 times/d for 2 d OR Famciclovir 125 mg bid for 5 d OR Valacyclovir 500 mg orally bid for 3 d OR Valacyclovir 1 g orally once daily for 5 d
Mpox	Mpox PCR lesion Mpox PCR rectal	Treatment: Oral tecovirimat (Tpoxx) https://www.cdc.gov/poxvirus/mpox/clinicians/obtaining-tecovirimat.html. Other treatment may be indicated if failure to respond to treatment, host factors, or tecovirimat contraindicated[53] https://www.cdc.gov/poxvirus/mpox/clinicians/treatment.html#anchor_1655488233196 Supportive care Pain management: • Stool softeners to reduce pain with bowel movements • Warm sitz baths (warm bath made up of water and baking soda or Epsom salt) • Oral acetaminophen or nonsteroidal anti-inflammatory drugs, topical anesthetics (eg, topical lidocaine), adjunctive pain relief with neuropathic pain agents, that is, gabapentin Antibiotics: to cover secondary bacterial infections if progressive erythema, pain, or swelling Itching: oral antihistamines, topical colloidals, topical calamine lotion, topical petroleum jelly Advanced disease[53]: refer for hospitalization; consult with infectious diseases; may require advanced specialty care

Abbreviations: ab/Ag, antibody/antigen; IgE, immunoglobulin E.
[a] Primary regimen also covers *N meningitidis*.
[b] The diagnosis of syphilis requires both a treponemal and a nontreponemal test (see Gilliams and colleagues in this issue for additional details on syphilis serologies).

There are several primary prevention tools in the armamentarium of STI and HIV prevention,[1] which may help clients guard against pathogens that may be associated with proctitis or HIV, a pathogen which may exacerbate it. These primary prevention tools include STI preexposure prophylaxis to prevent the acquisition of syphilis and CT, has been piloted, and is pending further study.[47] Doxycycline postexposure prophylaxis has been found to be effective in preventing bacterial STIs, including syphilis and

CT in MSM.[48] In a recent study in a US cohort of MSM and transgender women, effect was seen for CT, syphilis, and NG.[49] However, concerns were raised surrounding tetracycline resistance for NG and methicillin-resistant *Staphylococcus aureus*, highlighting the need to study this intervention in real-world settings (outside of clinical trials).[49] When it comes to prevention of enteric pathogens, such as *Shigella* spp, a mix of interventions may be needed. Behavioral counseling on the avoidance of sex when symptomatic or when partner is symptomatic of diarrheal disease, use of barrier protection, anogenital hygiene, substance use counseling and referrals, and tools to prevent HIV transmission are a few items to consider incorporating routinely in patient counseling.[8] Decreasing community HIV transmission by assuring equitable access to HIV postexposure prophylaxis, HIV preexposure prophylaxis, and rapid HIV treatment initiation and linkage to care are key for these bacterial STIs as well as Mpox. In addition, primary prevention through vaccination against pathogens associated with proctitis, such NM[22,50] and Mpox,[51,52] are important interventions to promote.

Last, incorporating partner services to reduce the likelihood of STI transmission in sexual networks, such as prevention counseling, STI screening, and treatment, is extremely important.[1] Use of public health staff, such as disease investigation services and application technologies (ie, anonymous partner notification tools), may allow us to get persons into care sooner to test, treat, and decrease STI transmission. Although acknowledging that in-person care visits for comprehensive evaluations and counseling may be best in populations where STI prevalence is high, it may not always be practical. Thus, for persons who are unable to present for care who are a contact to an STI, expedited partner therapy, where permissive in the United States, can be used.[1]

SUMMARY

Improved understanding of epidemiology, clinical manifestations, and pathogen profile of infectious proctitis is needed. Although STI care settings where extragenital testing is available offer testing for NG and CT infections, it is important to identify other potential causes, including MG, herpes, LGV, and syphilis. Furthermore, in this era of antimicrobial resistance concerns, availability of gonococcal susceptibility testing and MG macrolide resistance mutation assay would assist in antimicrobial stewardship. However, there remain knowledge gaps associated with the cause, risk factors, and clinical presentation associated with acquisition. Understanding behavioral risk and harm reduction conversations during clinical encounters should be implemented. Expanding our knowledge of the population-wide impact of vaccination programs targeting sexually transmissible pathogens and doxyPEP for STI prevention are needed. Emerging multipurpose prevention technologies for STIs/HIV will be an important technological advancement and are currently being investigated. Community acceptability of the various prevention tools will also be necessary to influence the alarming trends in STI prevalence.

CLINICS CARE POINTS

- Addressing STI incidence will require a multifactorial patient centered approach that incorporates clinical interventions based on behavioral risk, behavioral modification, and judicious harm reduction.
- Understanding population health and risk, as well as application of new technologies and vaccines targeting STI pathogens will be part of any comprehensive control plan.

- Novel applications of existing resources, such as doxycycline PEP show promise, but should be explored broadly regarding community impact, community acceptance, and unintended long term consequences.
- A combination of both novel and existing strategies will be needed to address the alarming increase in STI prevalence.

DISCLOSURES

In the past 12 months, C.J. McNeil has received research grants or contracts from Centers for Disease Control and Prevention, BARDA, United States/GSK, Becton Dickinson (BD), Cepheid, United States, Gilead, Hologic, United States, National Institutes of Health, United States paid to Wake Forest University School of Medicine. C.J. McNeil is on the advisory board for Talis Biomedical. L.F. Barroso has received grants or contracts funding from the National Institutes of Health and the AIDS Malignancy Consortium paid to Wake Forest University School of Medicine. K. Workowski has received grants or contracts from Gilead, Abbvie, United States, Centers for Disease Control and Prevention, United States, National Institutes of Health paid to Emory University.

REFERENCES

1. Workowski KA, Bachmann LH, Chan PA, et al. Sexually transmitted infections treatment guidelines, 2021. MMWR Recomm Rep (Morb Mortal Wkly Rep) 2021;70(4):1–187.
2. Klausner JD, Kohn R, Kent C. Etiology of clinical proctitis among men who have sex with men. Clin Infect Dis 2004;38(2):300–2.
3. Kumbhakar R, Barbee LA, Berzkalns A, et al. Etiologies of proctitis at a sexual health clinic in Seattle, Washington From 2011 to 2021. Sex Transm Dis 2022; 49(12).
4. Chan PA, Robinette A, Montgomery M, et al. Extragenital infections caused by Chlamydia trachomatis and Neisseria gonorrhoeae: a review of the literature. Infect Dis Obstet Gynecol 2016;2016:5758387.
5. Chandra NL, Broad C, Folkard K, et al. Detection of Chlamydia trachomatis in rectal specimens in women and its association with anal intercourse: a systematic review and meta-analysis. Sex Transm Infect 2018;94(5):320–6.
6. Dukers-Muijrers NH, Schachter J, van Liere GAFS, et al. What is needed to guide testing for anorectal and pharyngeal Chlamydia trachomatis and Neisseria gonorrhoeae in women and men? Evidence and opinion. BMC Infect Dis 2015; 15:533.
7. Pathela P, Blank S, Schillinger JA. Lymphogranuloma venereum: old pathogen, new story. Curr Infect Dis Rep 2007;9(2):143–50.
8. McNeil CJ, Kirkcaldy RD, Workowski K. Enteric infections in men who have sex with men. Clin Infect Dis 2022;74(Suppl_2):S169–78.
9. de Voux A, Kent JB, Macomber K, et al. Notes from the field: cluster of lymphogranuloma venereum cases among men who have sex with men - Michigan, 2016. MMWR Morb Mortal Wkly Rep 2016;65(34):920–1.
10. Pathela P, Jamison K, Kornblum J, et al. Lymphogranuloma venereum: an increasingly common anorectal infection among men who have sex with men attending New York City sexual health clinics. Sex Transm Dis 2019;46(2).

11. Peine B, Ved KJ, Fleming T, et al. Syphilitic proctitis presenting as locally advanced rectal cancer: a case report. Int J Surg Case Rep 2023;107:108358.
12. Costales-Cantrell JK, Dong EY, Wu BU, et al. Syphilitic proctitis presenting as a rectal mass: a case report and review of the literature. J Gen Intern Med 2021; 36(4):1098–101.
13. Ferzacca E, Barbieri A, Barakat L, et al. Lower gastrointestinal syphilis: case series and literature review. Open Forum Infect Dis 2021;8(6):ofab157.
14. Gutierrez-Fernandez J, Medina V, Hidalgo-Tenorio C, et al. Two Cases of Neisseria meningitidis Proctitis in HIV-positive men who have sex with men. Emerg Infect Dis 2017;23(3):542–3.
15. Bruzzesi E, Raccagni AR, Canetti D, et al. Proctitis and prostatitis by Neisseria meningitidis among MSM: A case series. J Infect 2022;85(2):174–211.
16. Read TRH, Murray GL, Danielewski JA, et al. Symptoms, sites, and significance of mycoplasma genitalium in men who have sex with men. Emerg Infect Dis 2019; 25(4):719–27.
17. Soni S, Alexander S, Verlander N, et al. The prevalence of urethral and rectal Mycoplasma genitalium and its associations in men who have sex with men attending a genitourinary medicine clinic. Sex Transm Infect 2010;86(1):21–4.
18. Francis SC, Kent CK, Klausner JD, et al. Prevalence of rectal Trichomonas vaginalis and Mycoplasma genitalium in male patients at the San Francisco STD clinic, 2005-2006. Sex Transm Dis 2008;35(9):797–800.
19. Chow EPF, Lee D, Bond S, et al. Nonclassical pathogens as causative agents of proctitis in men who have sex with men. Open Forum Infect Dis 2021;8(7): ofab137.
20. Ong JJ, Aung E, Read TRH, et al. Clinical characteristics of anorectal mycoplasma genitalium infection and microbial cure in men who have sex with men. Sex Transm Dis 2018;45(8):522–6.
21. Bissessor M, Fairley CK, Read T, et al. The etiology of infectious proctitis in men who have sex with men differs according to HIV status. Sex Transm Dis 2013; 40(10):768–70.
22. Adolescents, P.o.G.f.t.P.a.T.o.O.I.i.A.a., et al.
23. Kyaw NTT, Kipperman N, Alroy KA, et al. Notes from the field: clinical and epidemiologic characteristics of Mpox cases from the initial phase of the outbreak - New York City, May 19-July 15, 2022. MMWR Morb Mortal Wkly Rep 2022; 71(5152):1631–3.
24. Thornhill JP, Barkati S, Walmsley S, et al. Monkeypox virus infection in humans across 16 countries - april-june 2022. N Engl J Med 2022;387(8):679–91.
25. Rathore A, Kahn C, Reich D, et al. Monkeypox-induced proctitis: a case report of an emerging complication. Infection 2023;51(4):1165–8.
26. Yakubovsky M, Shasha D, Reich S, et al. Mpox presenting as proctitis in men who have sex with men. Clin Infect Dis 2023;76(3):528–30.
27. Shin H, Shin H, Rahmati M, et al. Comparison of clinical manifestations in mpox patients living with HIV versus without HIV: A systematic review and meta-analysis. J Med Virol 2023;95(4):e28713.
28. Curran KG, Eberly K, Russell OO, et al. HIV and sexually transmitted infections among persons with monkeypox - Eight U.S. Jurisdictions, May 17-July 22, 2022. MMWR Morb Mortal Wkly Rep 2022;71(36):1141–7.
29. Miller MJ, Cash-Goldwasser S, Marx GE, et al. Severe monkeypox in hospitalized patients - United States, August 10-October 10, 2022. MMWR Morb Mortal Wkly Rep 2022;71(44):1412–7.

30. Burdon RM, Atefi D, Rana J, et al. Sustained Mpox proctitis with primary syphilis and HIV seroconversion, Australia. Emerg Infect Dis 2023;29(3):647–9.
31. Jamard S, Handala L, Faussat C, et al. Resurgence of symptomatic Mpox among vaccinated patients: first clues from a new-onset local cluster. Infect Dis Now 2023;53(4):104714.
32. Faherty EAG, Holly T, Ogale YP, et al. Notes from the field: emergence of an Mpox cluster primarily affecting persons previously vaccinated against Mpox - Chicago, Illinois, March 18-June 12, 2023. MMWR Morb Mortal Wkly Rep 2023; 72(25):696–8.
33. Barrow RY, Ahmed F, Bolan GA, et al. Recommendations for providing quality sexually transmitted diseases clinical services, 2020. MMWR Recomm Rep (Morb Mortal Wkly Rep) 2020;68(5):1–20.
34. Davis TW, Goldstone SE. Sexually transmitted infections as a cause of proctitis in men who have sex with men. Dis Colon Rectum 2009;52(3):507–12.
35. Sonnenberg A. Age distribution of IBD hospitalization. Inflamm Bowel Dis 2010; 16(3):452–7.
36. London S, H.G., Tichauer MB. Anoscopy. Updated 2022 Aug 29.2023.
37. Palefsky JM, Lee JY, Jay N, et al. Treatment of anal high-grade squamous intraepithelial lesions to prevent anal cancer. N Engl J Med 2022;386(24):2273–82.
38. Palefsky JM. Practising high-resolution anoscopy. Sex Health 2012;9(6):580–6.
39. St Cyr S, Barbee L, Workowski KA, et al. Update to CDC's treatment guidelines for gonococcal infection, 2020. MMWR Morb Mortal Wkly Rep 2020;69(50): 1911–6.
40. Dombrowski JC, Wierzbicki MR, Newman LM, et al. Doxycycline Versus Azithromycin for the Treatment of Rectal Chlamydia in Men Who Have Sex With Men: A Randomized Controlled Trial. Clin Infect Dis 2021;73(5):824–31.
41. Lau A, Kong FYS, Fairley CK, et al. Azithromycin or Doxycycline for Asymptomatic Rectal Chlamydia trachomatis. N Engl J Med 2021;384(25):2418–27.
42. Simons R, Candfield S, French P, et al. Observed Treatment Responses to Short-Course Doxycycline Therapy for Rectal Lymphogranuloma Venereum in Men Who Have Sex With Men. Sex Transm Dis 2018;45(6):406–8.
43. Leeyaphan C, Ong JJ, Chow EPF, et al. Systematic Review and Meta-Analysis of Doxycycline Efficacy for Rectal Lymphogranuloma Venereum in Men Who Have Sex with Men. Emerg Infect Dis 2016;22(10):1778–84.
44. Liu HY, Han Y, Chen XS, et al. Comparison of efficacy of treatments for early syphilis: A systematic review and network meta-analysis of randomized controlled trials and observational studies. PLoS One 2017;12(6):e0180001.
45. Bachmann LH, Kirkcaldy RD, Geisler WM, et al. Prevalence of Mycoplasma genitalium Infection, Antimicrobial Resistance Mutations, and Symptom Resolution Following Treatment of Urethritis. Clin Infect Dis 2020;71(10):e624–32.
46. Manhart LE, Leipertz G, Soge OO, et al. Mycoplasma genitalium in the US (MyGeniUS): Surveillance Data from Sexual Health Clinics in Four US Regions. Clin Infect Dis 2023.
47. Bolan RK, Beymer MR, Weiss RE, et al. Doxycycline prophylaxis to reduce incident syphilis among HIV-infected men who have sex with men who continue to engage in high-risk sex: a randomized, controlled pilot study. Sex Transm Dis 2015;42(2):98–103.
48. Molina JM, Charreau I, Chidiac C, et al. Post-exposure prophylaxis with doxycycline to prevent sexually transmitted infections in men who have sex with men: an open-label randomised substudy of the ANRS IPERGAY trial. Lancet Infect Dis 2018;18(3):308–17.

49. Luetkemeyer AF, Donnell D, Dombrowski JC, et al. Postexposure doxycycline to prevent bacterial sexually transmitted infections. N Engl J Med 2023;388(14): 1296–306.
50. Mbaeyi SA, Duffy J, et al. Meningococcal vaccination: recommendations of the advisory committee on immunization practices, United States, 2020. MMWR Recomm Rep (Morb Mortal Wkly Rep) 2020;69(No. RR-9):1–41.
51. Rosenberg ES, Dorabawila V, Hart-Malloy R, et al. Effectiveness of JYNNEOS vaccine against diagnosed mpox infection - new york, 2022. MMWR Morb Mortal Wkly Rep 2023;72(20):559–63.
52. Dalton AF, Diallo AO, Chard AN, et al. Estimated effectiveness of JYNNEOS vaccine in preventing mpox: a multijurisdictional case-control study - united states, august 19, 2022-march 31, 2023. MMWR Morb Mortal Wkly Rep 2023;72(20): 553–8.
53. Rao AK, Schrodt CA, Minhaj FS, et al. Interim clinical treatment considerations for severe manifestations of mpox - united states, february 2023. MMWR Morb Mortal Wkly Rep 2023;72(9):232–43.

Update on Mpox

What the Primary Care Clinician Should Know

Jacob McLean, DO*, Shauna Gunaratne, MD, MPH, DTM&H,
Jason Zucker, MD, MS

KEYWORDS

• Mpox • Sexually transmitted infection • HIV • Emerging infectious disease

KEY POINTS

- Mpox is caused by a viral pathogen in the genus Orthopoxvirus related to the virus that causes smallpox.
- The 2022 outbreak has disproportionately affected men who have sex with men (MSM) and people with human immunodeficiency virus.
- Manifestations include a characteristic rash with or without systemic prodrome, and frequent anogenital involvement.
- Differential diagnosis is based on clinical syndrome and consists mainly of other sexually transmitted infections.
- Vaccination is available both as primary and postexposure prophylaxis and is critical to preventing epidemic resurgence.

BACKGROUND AND EPIDEMIOLOGY

The 2022 mpox epidemic transformed a previously neglected disease endemic to Western and Central Africa into a significant international concern. Mpox is a syndrome caused by the monkeypox virus (MPXV), a member of the Orthopoxvirus genus within the Poxviridae family.[1] MPXV was first isolated and described in 1958 by researchers in Denmark, who named the virus monkeypox due to the first known host, but this notably does not correlate with the animal reservoir for the disease, which is unknown.[2–5]

Two different MPXV clades have been identified; Clade I and Clade II, which is composed of 2 different subclades designated IIa and IIb.[6] In a mouse model, clade I seems to be most virulent (and is reported to cause up to 10% mortality in humans), with clade IIb as the least virulent.[7] Clade IIb virus has driven most cases in the 2022 outbreak.[6,7]

The first known human mpox case was described in 1970 in the Democratic Republic of the Congo in a 9-month-old infant.[8] Subsequent outbreaks have occurred primarily in West and Central Africa, with increasing frequency and case counts after the 1970s.[9] It

Division of Infectious Diseases, Columbia University Medical Center, 630 W 168th Street, Suite 876, New York, NY 10032, USA
* Corresponding author.
E-mail address: jm5146@cumc.columbia.edu

Med Clin N Am 108 (2024) 355–371
https://doi.org/10.1016/j.mcna.2023.09.005
medical.theclinics.com

is suspected that as smallpox immunity waned with decreasing vaccination campaigns, the number of mpox outbreaks increased in a population more susceptible to orthopoxviruses.[10]The first major outbreak of mpox in the western hemisphere took place in the United States in 2003, when 47 human cases were reported after contact with domesticated prairie dogs infected with MPXV from imported Ghanaian rodents.[11–13] There were no cases of human-to-human transmission.[12,13]

The first confirmed case in the 2022 outbreak dated to May 6, 2022, in the United Kingdom, followed by several cases that were unrelated to the first case and without recent travel history, indicating local transmission of MPXV.[3] Cases went on to be reported worldwide, prompting the WHO to declare mpox a global health emergency on July 23, 2022.[14,15]

Within the United States, the first identified case was reported on May 17, 2022. Incidence increased rapidly, peaking in August 2022, with nearly 700 cases per day. From October 2022 Centers for Disease Control (CDC) data, the median age of those diagnosed with mpox was 34 years. In patients with available data, 95% of cases were men, of whom 75% reported sexual contact with another man in the last 21 days. In the cases with known human immunodeficiency virus (HIV) status (only 20% of total cases), 57% cases had mpox and HIV coinfection.[16] As of this writing, there have been more than 87,500 cases worldwide, with 147 deaths. More than 85,900 cases were in areas that have not previously had mpox cases. The United States has contributed the bulk of cases with more than 30,000, followed by Brazil with nearly 11,000 and Spain with more than 7500.[17]

After August 2022, mpox incidence steadily declined, leading the US Department of Health and Human Services to allow the mpox public health emergency to expire on January 31, 2023,[18] with the WHO following suit on May 11, 2023.[19] The decrease in cases was likely driven by a combination of factors including behavioral changes[20] and immunity due to both vaccination and natural infection.[21] In the spring of 2023, however, a resurgence of mpox was observed in Chicago, Illinois, with 13 cases reported between April 17 and May 5, 2023. Notably, 69% of these were previously fully vaccinated against mpox.[21,22] The European Center for Disease Prevention and Control has also reported an increase of cases in April and early May 2023 with 17 new cases across 8 countries.[14]

TRANSMISSION

Transmission of the current epidemic of MPXV Clade IIb is thought be primarily through close physical contact, such as occurs during sexual activity. In the initial international case series by Thornhill and colleagues, skin and anogenital lesions had the highest rate of positivity (97%), with much lower rates in samples from the nasopharynx (26%), blood (7%), and urine (3%).[23] Further reports have suggested higher MPXV loads in genital, skin lesion, and rectal samples than in those from pharyngeal, urine, blood, or nasopharyngeal samples, demonstrating more inefficient respiratory transmission.[24,25] Viral DNA is shed for up to 3 weeks after symptom onset, although some studies have shown low-level detectable DNA for longer periods.[26] In one cohort study from Spain, replication-competent virus was found only in the first 21 days at any body site, with skin lesions having the highest viral loads and longest duration of replication-competent virus.[27] No MPXV transmissions have been observed after lesions have healed. Presymptomatic transmission has been reported up to 4 days before symptom onset.[26]

Household Transmission to Children

Household transmission to children has been rare in the United States during this outbreak. In a case series from California, the overall rate of mpox in children was low, representing only 0.3% cases in California. The MPXV calculated secondary attack rate was 4.7%.[28]

Health Care-associated Transmission

Overall HCP acquisition rates seem low—in a report published on Colorado health-care personnel (HCP) exposed to mpox, there were 0 cases of mpox despite overall low rates (23%) of adherence to recommended personal protective equipment.[29] This is also consistent with earlier outbreaks, where the rate of transmission to HCP is extremely low, with only 1 case reported before the 2022 outbreak.[30] The greatest risk of mpox transmission to HCP seems to be with needlestick injuries from equipment used to unroof vesicles or lesions.[31–35]

CLINICAL PRESENTATION

Until the 2022 outbreak, descriptions of the mpox clinical syndrome were drawn from a relatively few endemic and epidemic case series. In this context, the initial symptom in most infected individuals was a systemic prodrome consisting of fever, headache, myalgias, malaise, and lymphadenopathy, which was then followed by the development of a characteristic rash. Skin lesions were typically described as disseminated and synchronous, progressing through stages from macule, to papule, vesicle, pustule, and then scab.[36,37]

The recent outbreak has been notable for key differences in presentation. Rash has been the *initial* symptom in approximately half of patients and can be asynchronous. Most patients will, however, experience at least one systemic symptom at some time during the course of their infection.[38–41] Generalized lymphadenopathy may be present during prodrome but localized lymphadenopathy is more common.

Lesions can exist in any of the stages noted above, with frequent umbilication in the papular/pustular stage (**Fig. 1**). They are typically painful, especially entering the papular phase, and can become pruritic as they scab and heal. Most individuals have involvement of the oral and/or anogenital areas, with or without affected skin at other sites including the palms and soles. Most have fewer than 20 lesions at presentation and, importantly, cases have been reported of mucosal infection *without* visible skin lesions.

Mucosal involvement is common and may reflect the site(s) of exposure. In a case series from the 2022 outbreak, proctitis was noted in approximately 20% to 30% of mpox cases[42–44] and was a frequent driver of hospital admission.[45,46] Proctitis typically presents with anorectal pain, tenesmus, and discharge with or without diarrhea *or* constipation. External lesions around the anus may or may not be visible. Sore

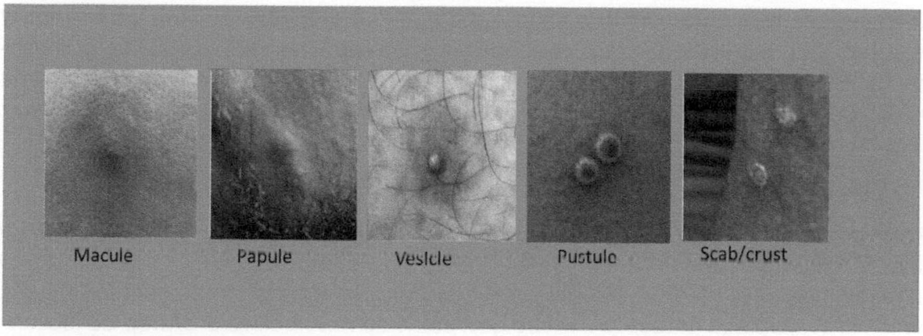

Fig. 1. Stages of mpox lesions.

throat may occur as part of the systemic infectious syndrome but direct oropharyngeal mucosal involvement is also relatively common. The least frequent but potentially most morbid mucosal manifestation is ocular infection, which can include conjunctivitis, blepharitis, or keratitis.[47–49]

Immunocompromised individuals can develop more severe manifestations, including high-burden skin and mucosal lesions, as well as other organ involvement such as pneumonia or encephalitis. Notably, individuals with well-controlled HIV present with similar symptoms and disease severity as those without HIV.[45] In all individuals, lesions may develop bacterial superinfection with resulting ulceration and/or cellulitis.

Laboratory abnormalities occur frequently and are nonspecific, including cytopenias (especially lymphopenia), thrombocytosis, and transaminase elevation.

DIFFERENTIAL DIAGNOSIS

Earlier literature regarding differential diagnoses for mpox relied primarily on differentiating this infection from smallpox, with mpox distinguished by the presence of lymphadenopathy and synchronous skin lesions. In the postsmallpox era, mpox differential diagnosis hinges on the clinical syndromes and risk groups noted above. Differential diagnoses based on clinical syndrome are reported in **Table 1**, along with differentiating characteristics for each pathogen.

As rash is present in almost all patients with mpox, this directs the primary differential diagnosis, with each alternative agent having distinct rash characteristics. Herpes Simplex Virus (HSV) and Varicella Zoster Virus (VZV) can resemble the vesicular lesions of mpox, and molluscum contagiosum the more umbilicated stage, whereas secondary syphilis can cause a diffuse rash (which is classically macular but can be pustular or ulcerative) accompanied by systemic symptoms. Finally, although rash is a less-common presentation, HIV should be ruled out in all individuals presenting with the symptoms above and relevant epidemiologic risk.

Individuals presenting with genital ulcer disease should additionally be considered for diagnoses of HSV, syphilis, chancroid, and lymphogranuloma venereum (LGV). Genital herpes (HSV) in particular can be difficult to distinguish from mpox, with earlier episodes being the primary clue on history, and nucleic acid amplification testing (NAAT) testing being the only way to definitively distinguish these.

Chlamydia (including LGV), gonorrhea, HSV, and syphilis should also be part of the differential diagnosis for individuals with proctitis. Proctocolitis, in which individuals develop abdominal pain and diarrhea in addition to rectal pain, tenesmus, and discharge can be caused by LGV as well as enteric organisms such as *Salmonella*, *Shigella*, and *Campylobacter*, especially among MSM.[50]

All patients suspected of mpox should undergo comprehensive sexually transmitted infection (STI) testing regardless of specific symptoms. This should include, at a minimum, HIV antibody/antigen testing, syphilis serologies, and gonorrhea/chlamydia NAAT from the rectum, pharynx, and urine/cervix as indicated.

TESTING/DIAGNOSIS

Polymerase chain reaction (PCR) analysis of specimens obtained from infected body sites is the primary means of confirming a diagnosis of mpox. The CDC has published a helpful guide for medical professionals collecting specimens to be sent for testing, which is available at (https://www.cdc.gov/poxvirus/mpox/clinicians/prep-collection-specimens.html). Serology is not routinely used.

Table 1
Differential diagnoses of mpox-related syndromes and distinguishing features of other pathogens

Syndrome	Common Infectious Differentials	Distinguishing Features
Rash (localized or general)		
	HSV	• History of earlier outbreaks • Generalized rash less common • Systemic symptoms uncommon with localized rash
	VZV	• Dermatomal distribution (shingles) • Isolated anogenital involvement less common
	Molluscum contagiosum	• Lesions typically painless • Systemic symptoms, mucosal involvement, and lesions on palms/soles less common
	Secondary syphilis	• Rash lacks vesicles or umbilication, although can be ulcerated or pustular
	Acute HIV	• Umbilication of skin lesions and anogenital involvement are uncommon
Genital ulcer		
	HSV	• History of earlier outbreaks • Systemic symptoms are rare
	Primary syphilis	• Typically painless
	Lymphogranuloma venereum	• Ulcer typically painless, often resolved at time of presentation
	Chancroid	• Currently rare in the United States
Proctitis		
	Gonorrhea	• No papular/vesicular lesions • No systemic symptoms
	Chlamydia (serovars D-K)	• No papular/vesicular lesions • No systemic symptoms
	Lymphogranuloma venereum	• Genital ulcer typically not concurrent with proctitis
	Secondary syphilis	• Can present with rectal mass but genital ulcers are generally not concurrent
	HSV	• History of earlier outbreaks
	Enteric bacteria	• No ulcers or skin/mucosal lesions

Skin lesions are the recommended source of specimens and can comprise swabs of intact lesions or exudate, as well as samples of crust. At least 2 lesions from different body sites and different stages should be sampled, with 2 swabs sent per lesion. Swabs should be made from a synthetic material such as nylon or Dacron—*not* cotton. Both dry swabs and viral transport media can be used but bacterial transport media should be avoided as these can interfere with the PCR assay. It is important to confirm the exact swab/transport media requirement with the laboratory processing the specimen before testing. Requirements for specimens sent to the CDC can be found at the URL above.

Once mpox is suspected, and before swabbing lesions, the CDC recommends that providers don appropriate personal protective equipment, defined as gown, gloves, eye protection, and a respirator (eg, N95) mask. Swabs should be held in such a way that the gloved fingers do not touch any part of the final specimen—for swabs transported in liquid media, this means holding the swab above the portion that will ultimately be submerged. Swabs should be pressed firmly against the lesion and swiped back and forth, with this process repeated on the other side of the swab. Unroofing lesions is not recommended because this is not required for an adequate sample and incurs a risk of needle-stick injury and iatrogenic infection. If accepted by the laboratory handling the specimen, crusts at least 4 mm × 4 mm can be removed with forceps or another sterile instrument and transported in a dry, sterile container.

If a patient has no skin lesions, but mpox is still suspected, virus has been successfully detected at other sites including oropharyngeal and rectal mucosa as well as urine, although this testing is neither currently the Food and Drug Administration (FDA)-approved nor available from commercial laboratories.[51] At least one study has shown that testing one of these other sites in *addition* to skin lesions does not increase diagnostic yield.[52]

All laboratories performing mpox testing should report positive results to the applicable local health department. In order to report suspected mpox clinicians can contact their state health department or the CDC Emergency Operations Center at (770-488-7100).

TRANSMISSION PRECAUTIONS

People with mpox who do not require hospitalization should make every attempt to limit contact with others to prevent the spread of the virus. Ideally, this would be isolation at home in an area separated from other individuals but this may not always be practical. The CDC recommends that individuals with mpox avoid close, skin-to-skin contact including sexual contact until all lesions have healed completely and all other symptoms have resolved. Crowds and congregate settings should be avoided when possible, and clothes, gloves, and/or bandages should cover all skin lesions when in shared spaces. Items that may have come into contact with infected lesions or mucosa, such as clothes, towels, bedding, and eating or drinking utensils, should not be shared. These items should be washed or disinfected before being used by other individuals. The CDC additionally recommends that people with mpox wear a well-fitting mask when in close contact with others, although the role of respiratory transmission in the recent outbreak remains unclear. Additional caution should be taken to avoid contact with high-risk individuals including immunocompromised people. People with mpox and those around them can be reassured that brief contact such as a short conversation, or even prolonged proximity without physical contact has not been shown to spread mpox.[53]

PROGNOSIS

Fortunately, the course of mpox is self-limited in most cases; according to CDC statistics, the United States' case fatality rate for mpox was 1.3 per 1000 cases. However, this statistical changes dramatically among immunosuppressed individuals. Nearly 94% of US deaths due to mpox occurred among people with HIV, and among the subset of those with available data, all had CD4 counts less than 200.[54]

Although most survivors experience no long-term sequelae, scarring at lesion sites has been reported and can be of cosmetic concern in areas such as the face or genitals.[55] Concern has also been raised for risk of strictures of the anus or urethra.

The timeline of mpox recovery varies based on severity, and illness can be prolonged among those with severe disease and especially immunosuppression. For most individuals, however, the total course of illness is approximately 2 to 4 weeks, and nearly all patients can expect to make a full recovery.

POSTEXPOSURE PROPHYLAXIS

Individuals with exposure to mpox should be offered a dose of mpox vaccine as postexposure prophylaxis. Vaccination is recommended within 4 days for optimal efficacy but receipt of vaccine between 4 and 14 days may also confer some degree of protection. Those who do not go on to develop symptomatic infection should complete the full 2-dose vaccine series. Thus far, evidence for this practice is limited to the use of smallpox vaccine in 30 exposed individuals during the much smaller 2003 US mpox outbreak, with only 1 subsequent symptomatic infection.[56] Although efforts are underway to evaluate this strategy during the 2022 outbreak,[57] public data regarding efficacy is not yet available. Some clinics may have the capacity to keep mpox vaccine on hand for both primary and postexposure prophylaxis. In cases where this is not feasible, primary care providers should contact their local health department regarding vaccine availability.

PRIMARY PREVENTION

Vaccination efforts have been central to containing the recent mpox outbreak. The principal vaccine currently in use is based on Modified Vaccinia Ankara (MVA), a live but replication-deficient virus strain developed in the late stages of the global campaign to eradicate smallpox. Unlike earlier smallpox vaccines such ACAM2000 or Dryvax, vaccines based on MVA are *not* capable of causing infection. Of note, vaccines based on this virus are not a recent development—one was deployed in Germany in the 1970s as a primer for other smallpox vaccines, where it was administered to more than 100,000 people with an excellent safety profile.[58] The currently available product in the United States is manufactured by Bavarian Nordic under the trade name JYNNEOS.

Mpox vaccine is administered as a 2-dose series of either subcutaneous or intradermal injections spaced 4 weeks apart. Intradermal administration typically is performed on the volar surface of the forearm, and subcutaneous dosing over the tricep or deltoid (adults) or anterolateral thigh (children aged <12 years). Intradermal dosing has been favored during periods of limited vaccine supply due to the lower dose required, allowing for increased numbers of individuals to be vaccinated but only the subcutaneous route is FDA licensed at this time. Evidence for intradermal administration is based on studies showing comparable levels of resulting antibody titers but there is not yet clinical data comparing the 2 routes of administration.[59] At present, they are considered interchangeable.

At the time of publication, the CDC recommends mpox vaccination for primary prevention in groups at elevated risk of infection (**Box 1**). The full vaccination recommendations can be accessed at: https://www.cdc.gov/poxvirus/mpox/interim-considerations/overview.html.

Estimates of vaccine efficacy from restrospective data have ranged from 35.8% to 86% for 1 dose and 66% to 88.5% for 2 doses of vaccine.[60–64]

Vaccination side effects are rare.[65] Local reactions such as pain, erythema, swelling, or pruritis are the most common and can be managed with topical emollients, cold compresses, and/or oral antihistamines. Intradermal vaccination seems to confer a higher risk of local cutaneous adverse reaction, with erythema lasting only a few days[66] but subsequent hyperpigmentation that may be more prolonged.[67]

VACCINE EQUITY

The mpox epidemic has disproportionately affected GBMSM community and certain racial and ethnic groups. In the United States, the incidence of mpox was highest in

Box 1 Mpox vaccination (Modified Vaccinia Ankara)
Schedule 2 doses administered 28 d apart
Groups recommended for primary prevention • Gay and bisexual men who have sex with men with either: ◦ More than 1 sex partner in the last 6 months ◦ Any STI in the last 6 months • Individuals engaging in sex at a commercial sex venue or in association with a large public event • Sexual partners of individuals in the above groups • Individuals with immunosuppression (including HIV) who anticipate contact with mpox • Those with occupational risk, primarily laboratory workers
Postexposure prophylaxis • Preferably within 4 d of exposure, may offer some protection out to 14 d

Black and Hispanic men, with a relative risk (RR) of 6.9 in Black men and an RR of 4.1 in Hispanic men, when compared with White men. Unfortunately, vaccination rates were also lower in these groups, with the lowest vaccination-to-case ratios observed in Black men (8.8) and Hispanic men (16.2) compared with White men (42.5). Early in the outbreak, vaccination rates were lower in Black and Hispanic men than in White men, perhaps reflecting structural barriers to accessing vaccination when resources were limited. The disparity in vaccination-to-case ratios reflected the greater unmet vaccination needs in the groups most vulnerable to mpox infection.[68]

PROTECTION FROM EARLIER MPOX INFECTION OR SMALLPOX VACCINATION

Given the earlier widespread use of smallpox vaccine (discontinued in the United States in 1972), there has been considerable interest in ascertaining the degree of protection conferred by these earlier vaccine products. Cross-sectional studies from the Democratic Republic of Congo suggest that mpox incidence increased significantly after the discontinuation of routine smallpox vaccination and that previously vaccinated individuals had a lower risk of future mpox infection.[10,69] However, at least one study in the recent outbreak has failed to find any association between history of smallpox vaccine receipt and risk of infection.[43] At present, history of earlier smallpox vaccination should not be a factor in the decision to vaccinate against mpox.

The degree of protection conferred by earlier mpox infection is also currently unknown. At present, previously infected individuals are considered immune but there have now been several reported cases of potential reinfection.[70,71] The degree and durability of infection conferred by earlier infection, as well as the effect of immune compromise on these parameters, remains to be established.

MANAGEMENT CONSIDERATIONS

Most patients with mpox achieve full recovery, regardless of whether they receive treatment or not. Although the FDA has not approved any therapies specifically for mpox, supportive care measures have been used for pain control while medications initially developed for smallpox treatment have been reutilized as medical countermeasures (**Table 2**). These countermeasures may be beneficial for patients who are at risk for severe disease such as those who are immunocompromised, those with severe disease, and those with lesions in areas that might result in serious sequelae, for example, the eye

Table 2
Mpox treatment

Location of Lesions	Proctitis	Oropharyngeal Lesions	Skin and Genital Lesions
Supportive care	Stool softeners Lidocaine gel Sitz baths Anti-inflammatories Opioids	Antiseptic mouthwash Viscous lidocaine Saltwater gargles Anti-inflammatories Opioids	Wash with gentle emollients Apply petroleum jelly to skin lesions Consider DuoDERM dressing for persistent lesions Antibiotics if required for bacterial superinfection
Medical Countermeasures	Indication		Standard Dosing
Tecovirimat	First line for those with severe disease or at risk for severe disease. Available through clinical trials or EA-IND		600 mg PO or IV twice daily (3 × daily for those >120 kg) for 14 d
Brincidofovir Cidofovir	Second-line therapy for those who cannot receive tecovirimat, side effect profiles may determine which drug to choose. One animal study suggests that combined treatment with tecovirimat might be synergistic and is an option for individuals with severe or progressive disease		200 mg PO weekly × 2 wk 5 mg/kg IV weekly × 2 wk
VIGIV	Individuals unable or unlikely to mount a robust immune response (immunocompromised due to disease or medications)		6–9000 units/kg IV once
Trifluridine	Individuals with ocular disease		One drop every 2 h × 2 wk

or urethra. Nonetheless, no medications have been definitively proven effective in randomized controlled trials. The CDC maintains a clinical guidance resource page for clinicians addressing both supportive care as well as medical countermeasures at https://www.cdc.gov/poxvirus/mpox/clinicians/clinical-guidance.html. Patients requiring medical countermeasures should be managed in consultation with infectious diseases specialists and/or local health authorities. See **Fig. 2** for suggested workflow for the initial evaluation of mpox in the primary care setting.

Supportive Care Guidelines

Recommendations for supportive care primarily derive from expert consensus. In the case of proctitis, stool softeners can help reduce pain during defecation while topical therapies such as sitz baths and lidocaine gels may offer additional comfort. Caution is advised when using topical steroids due to the risk of local immunosuppression. Over-the-counter analgesics such as nonsteroidal anti-inflammatory drugs or acetaminophen are often adequate, although prescription pain relievers such as gabapentin or opioids have been used for some patients with severe pain. For those experiencing pharyngeal disease, viscous lidocaine and saltwater gargles can provide additional relief. Finally, considering that secondary bacterial infection is a possible complication, antibiotics should be considered when bacterial superinfection is suspected.[72,73]

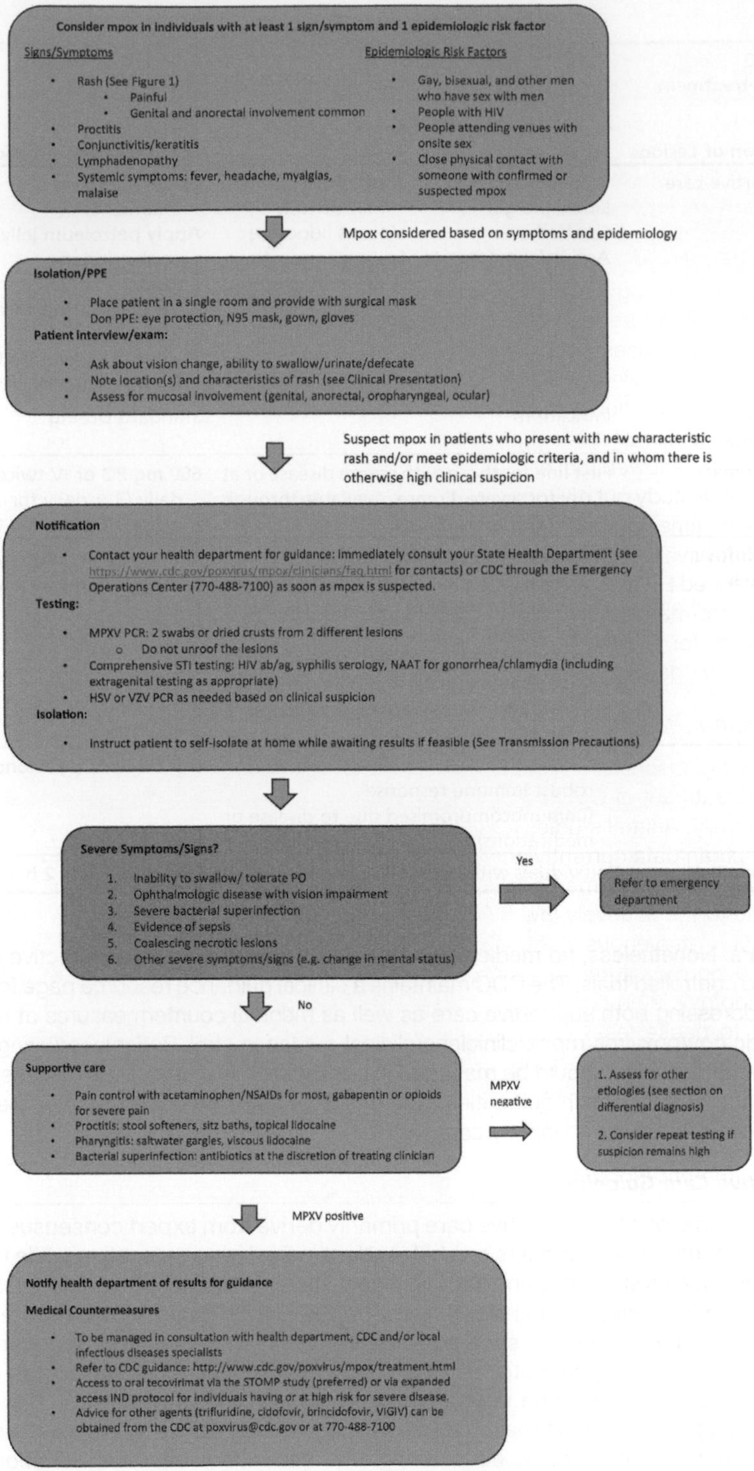

Fig. 2. Suggested workflow for mpox in the primary care setting. CDC, Centers for Disease Control; PO, oral intake.

Tecovirimat

Tecovirimat is an antiviral medication originally engineered to treat variola virus for the treatment of smallpox. Its mechanism of action involves inhibiting viral protein p37, a target that is highly specific and conserved across orthopoxviruses. The FDA approved tecovirimat in 2018 under the Animal Efficacy Rule, a regulation permitting drug approval for severe or life-threatening conditions where human efficacy trials are neither ethical nor practical. Before the recent outbreak, only human safety studies were accessible.[74]

For those needing treatment during the 2022 outbreak, tecovirimat became first-line treatment, with more than 6800 courses administered across the United States via a CDC expanded access investigational new drug (EA-IND) protocol.[75,76] Although safety data are encouraging, there is currently no randomized controlled human efficacy data.[77] An observational study of 154 patients receiving tecovirimat showed that HIV status did not affect clinical presentations or treatment results.[45] However, a report from the CDC showed that all 27 mpox-associated fatalities had been treated with tecovirimat and a study out of Rome found no evidence of large effect of tecovirimat in healing time or time to viral clearance in a small hospitalized population.[54,78] Given the limited data available, tecovirimat, through a clinical trial, should be offered to patients with advanced HIV or severe disease, with the EA-IND available to those unable to enroll in a trial. Information about how to access tecovirimat through the clinical trial Study of Tecovirimat for Human Monkeypox Virus (STOMP) or the EA-IND can be found at https://www.cdc.gov/poxvirus/mpox/clinicians/obtaining-tecovirimat.html.

Cidofovir/Brincidofovir

Cidofovir diphosphate is a competitive inhibitor of DNA polymerase, approved by the FDA for treatment of CMV retinitis. Cidofovir can be used topically, intralesionally, or intravenously. Animal studies point to potential effectiveness against orthopoxviruses but no human data currently confirms its efficacy in treating mpox. Case studies suggest possible improvements following intravenous cidofovir administration[79,80]; however, due to the relatively low mortality rate of this disease and the substantial risk of renal injury, intravenous cidofovir has been mainly used for individuals with severe disease and significant immunosuppression.

Brincidofovir is an oral prodrug of cidofovir available through an EA-IND, which is thought to cause less renal toxicity but that may induce hepatotoxicity.[50] Animal studies suggest that the combination of tecovirimat and brincidofovir may act synergistically.[81] This pairing should be contemplated for patients with severe immunosuppression and progressive disease.

Vaccinia Immunoglobulin

The passive transfer of antibodies against the vaccinia virus is presumed to provide cross-protection against mpox and vaccinia immunoglobulin (VIGIV), and may provide additional beneficial immunocompromised individuals, particularly those with advanced HIV. Case reports indicate improvement following this therapy, suggesting that VIGIV should be evaluated in patients with advanced HIV and severe mpox.[82]

Trifluridine Drops

Trifluridine drops, which are FDA-approved for the treatment of herpes simplex virus eye infections, are thought to have activity against orthopoxviruses.[49,83–85] They should be considered for all patients with ocular disease.

SUMMARY

The 2022 outbreak was the most widespread epidemic of mpox to date, significant not only for large case numbers but also for the disproportionate burden of disease among men who have sex with men and people with HIV. At the time of writing, incidence is low but there remains significant risk of resurgence within communities where immunity from vaccination or earlier infection is low.[86] Differentiating mpox from other infections will depend in part on current disease dynamics—providers should stay abreast of their local epidemiology. Continued efforts to vaccinate at-risk individuals are critical to avoiding further instances of generalized transmission. Treatment remains primarily supportive given the self-limited nature of disease. Antiviral therapy, particularly with tecovirimat, shows promise but should ideally be undertaken in the context of a clinical trial because there is not yet definitive proof of efficacy.

CLINICS CARE POINTS

- Primary prevention with vaccination is effective and should be offered to all at-risk individuals
- Postexposure prophylaxis using the mpox vaccine may avert infection or shorten symptom duration/severity
- Individuals with suspected or confirmed mpox should receive comprehensive STI screening
- Individuals with suspected or confirmed mpox should self-isolate at home when possible and avoid close physical contact until all symptoms/lesions have resolved
- Local or state health departments should be notified of new cases of confirmed mpox
- Supportive care is the mainstay of treatment, consisting of topical and/or systemic analgesia as well as treatment of bacterial superinfection and co-occurring STIs if present
- For individuals with severe disease, consultation should be sought with a local infectious disease expert and/or the CDC
- Medical countermeasures are available for individuals with severe disease. Individuals with or without severe disease can be enrolled in STOMP, an efficacy study of the antiviral medication tecovirimat

FUNDING

NIH, United States 5T32AI100852-10 (JM), NIAID, United States K23AI150378 (JZ)

DISCLOSURE

The authors report no commercial or financial conflicts of interest.

REFERENCES

1. Ulaeto D, Agafonov A, Burchfield J, et al. New nomenclature for mpox (monkeypox) and monkeypox virus clades. Lancet Infect Dis 2023;23(3):273–5.
2. Elsayed S, Bondy L, Hanage WP. Monkeypox Virus Infections in Humans. Clin Microbiol Rev 2022;35(4):e0009222.
3. Gessain A, Nakoune E, Yazdanpanah Y. Monkeypox. New England Journal of Medicine 2022;387(19):1783–93. https://doi.org/10.1056/NEJMra2208860.
4. Magnus PV, Andersen EK, Petersen KB, et al. A pox-like disease in cynomolgus monkeys. Acta Pathol Microbiol Scand 1959;46(2):156–76.

5. Damaso CR. Phasing out monkeypox: mpox is the new name for an old disease. Lancet Regional Health - Americas 2023;17:100424.
6. Happi C, Adetifa I, Mbala P, et al. Urgent need for a non-discriminatory and non-stigmatizing nomenclature for monkeypox virus. PLoS Biol 2022;20(8):e3001769.
7. Americo JL, Earl PL, Moss B. Virulence differences of mpox (monkeypox) virus clades I, IIa, and IIb.1 in a small animal model. Proc Natl Acad Sci USA 2023; 120(8). e2220415120.
8. Ladnyj ID, Ziegler P, Kima E. A human infection caused by monkeypox virus in Basankusu Territory, Democratic Republic of the Congo. Bull World Health Organ 1972;46(5):593–7.
9. Beer EM, Rao VB. A systematic review of the epidemiology of human monkeypox outbreaks and implications for outbreak strategy. PLoS Negl Trop Dis 2019; 13(10):e0007791.
10. Rimoin AW, Mulembakani PM, Johnston SC, et al. Major increase in human monkeypox incidence 30 years after smallpox vaccination campaigns cease in the Democratic Republic of Congo. Proc Natl Acad Sci USA 2010;107(37):16262–7.
11. Update: Multistate Outbreak of Monkeypox—Illinois, Indiana, Kansas, Missouri, Ohio, and Wisconsin, 2003. JAMA 2003;290(3):325. https://doi.org/10.1001/jama.290.3.325.
12. Cdc. Mpox in the U.S. Past U.S. Cases and outbreaks. Centers for Disease Control and Prevention; 2022.
13. Reynolds MG, Davidson WB, Curns AT, et al. Spectrum of Infection and Risk Factors for Human Monkeypox, United States, 2003. Emerg Infect Dis 2007;13(9): 1332–9.
14. Ecdc. Joint ECDC-WHO regional office for europe mpox surveillance bulletin. Joint ECDC-WHO Regional Office for Europe Mpox Surveillance Bulletin; 2023.
15. Organization WH. WHO Director-General's statement at the press conference following IHR Emergency Committee regarding the multi-country outbreak of monkeypox - 23 July 2022. Accessed June 10, 2023. https://www.who.int/director-general/speeches/detail/who-director-general-s-statement-on-the-press-conference-following-IHR-emergency-committee-regarding-the-multi–country-outbreak-of-monkeypox–23-july-2022.
16. Kava CM, Rohraff DM, Wallace B, et al. Epidemiologic Features of the Monkeypox Outbreak and the Public Health Response — United States, May 17–October 6, 2022. MMWR Morb Mortal Wkly Rep 2022;71(45):1449–56.
17. CDC. Mpox in the U.S. 2022 mpox outbreak global map. Centers for Disease Control and Prevention; 2023.
18. Services USDoHaH. Statement From HHS Secretary Becerra on mpox. Accessed Jun 10, 2023. https://www.hhs.gov/about/news/2022/12/02/statement-from-hhs-secretary-becerra-on-mpox.html.
19. Organization WH. Fifth Meeting of the International Health Regulations (2005) (IHR) Emergency Committee on the Multi-Country Outbreak of mpox (monkeypox). Accessed June 10, 2023. https://www.who.int/news/item/11-05-2023-fifth-meeting-of-the-international-health-regulations-(2005)-(ihr)-emergency-committee-on-the-multi-country-outbreak-of-monkeypox-(mpox).
20. Delaney KP, Sanchez T, Hannah M, et al. Strategies Adopted by Gay, Bisexual, and Other Men Who Have Sex with Men to Prevent Monkeypox virus Transmission - United States, August 2022. MMWR Morb Mortal Wkly Rep 2022;71(35): 1126–30.
21. Alert Detail - HAN - Chicago Health Alert Network. HAN.

22. Health Alert Network (HAN) - 00490 | Potential Risk for New Mpox Cases. 2023/05/15/T01:57:44Z 2023.
23. Thornhill JP, Barkati S, Walmsley S, et al. Monkeypox Virus Infection in Humans across 16 Countries - April-June 2022. N Engl J Med 2022;387(8):679–91.
24. MPOX VIRAL LOAD BY SPECIMEN TYPE AND DIAGNOSTIC TESTING IN A CLINICAL LABORATORY - CROI Conference. 2023. https://www.croiconference.org/abstract/mpox-viral-load-by-specimen-type-and-diagnostic-testing-in-a-clinical-laboratory/.
25. MPOX IN Amsterdam: CROSS-SECTIONAL STUDY AMONG MSM AT THE CENTRE FOR SEXUAL HEALTH - CROI Conference. 2023. https://www.croiconference.org/abstract/mpox-in-amsterdam-cross-sectional-study-among-msm-at-the-centre-for-sexual-health/.
26. Cdc. Mpox in the U.S. Science brief: detection and transmission of mpox (formerly monkeypox) virus during the 2022 clade IIb outbreak. Centers for Disease Control and Prevention; 2023.
27. Suñer C, Ubals M, Tarín-Vicente EJ, et al. Viral dynamics in patients with monkeypox infection: a prospective cohort study in Spain. Lancet Infect Dis 2023;23(4):445–53.
28. HOUSEHOLD TRANSMISSION OF MPOX TO CHILDREN AND ADOLESCENTS - CROI Conference. 2023. https://www.croiconference.org/abstract/household-transmission-of-mpox-to-children-and-adolescents/.
29. Marshall KE, Barton M, Nichols J, et al. Health Care Personnel Exposures to Subsequently Laboratory-Confirmed Monkeypox Patients — Colorado, 2022. MMWR Morb Mortal Wkly Rep 2022;71(38):1216–9.
30. Zachary KC, Shenoy ES. Monkeypox transmission following exposure in healthcare facilities in nonendemic settings: Low risk but limited literature. Infect Control Hosp Epidemiol 2022;43(7):920–4.
31. Caldas JP, Valdoleiros SR, Rebelo S, et al. Monkeypox after Occupational Needlestick Injury from Pustule. Emerg Infect Dis 2022;28(12). https://doi.org/10.3201/eid2812.221374.
32. Carvalho LB, Casadio LVB, Polly M, et al. Monkeypox Virus Transmission to Healthcare Worker through Needlestick Injury, Brazil. Emerg Infect Dis 2022;28(11):2334–6.
33. Le Pluart D, Ruyer-Thompson M, Ferré VM, et al. A Healthcare-Associated Infection With Monkeypox Virus of a Healthcare Worker During the 2022 Outbreak. Open Forum Infect Dis 2022;9(10):ofac520. https://doi.org/10.1093/ofid/ofac520.
34. Mendoza R, Petras JK, Jenkins P, et al. *Monkeypox Virus* Infection Resulting from an Occupational Needlestick — Florida, 2022. MMWR Morb Mortal Wkly Rep 2022;71(42):1348–9.
35. Choi Y, Jeon E-B, Kim T, et al. Case Report and Literature Review of Occupational Transmission of Monkeypox Virus to Healthcare Workers, South Korea. Emerg Infect Dis 2023;29(5):997–1001.
36. Titanji BK, Tegomoh B, Nematollahi S, et al. Monkeypox: A Contemporary Review for Healthcare Professionals. Open Forum Infect Dis 2022;9(7):ofac310.
37. Ogoina D, Iroezindu M, James HI, et al. Clinical Course and Outcome of Human Monkeypox in Nigeria. Clin Infect Dis 2020;71(8):e210–4.
38. Mailhe M, Beaumont AL, Thy M, et al. Clinical characteristics of ambulatory and hospitalized patients with monkeypox virus infection: an observational cohort study. Clin Microbiol Infect 2023;29(2):233–9.
39. Orviz E, Negredo A, Ayerdi O, et al. Monkeypox outbreak in Madrid (Spain): Clinical and virological aspects. J Infect 2022;85(4):412–7.

40. Philpott DHC, Alroy KA, Alroy KA, et al. Epidemiologic and clinical characteristics of monkeypox cases — United States, May 17–July 22, 2022. MMWR Morb Mortal Wkly Rep 2022;71:1018–22.
41. Centers for Disease Control and Prevention NCfEaZIDN, Division of High-Consequence Pathogens and Pathology (DHCPP). Science Brief: Detection and Transmission of Mpox (Formerly Monkeypox) Virus During the 2022 Clade IIb Outbreak. Accessed 5/10/23, https://www.cdc.gov/poxvirus/mpox/about/science-behind-transmission.html.
42. Cassir N, Cardona F, Tissot-Dupont H, et al. Observational cohort study of evolving epidemiologic, clinical, and virologic features of monkeypox in Southern France. Emerg Infect Dis 2022;28(12):2409–15.
43. Catala A, Clavo-Escribano P, Riera-Monroig J, et al. Monkeypox outbreak in Spain: clinical and epidemiological findings in a prospective cross-sectional study of 185 cases. Br J Dermatol 2022. https://doi.org/10.1111/bjd.21790.
44. Tarin-Vicente EJ, Alemany A, Agud-Dios M, et al. Clinical presentation and virological assessment of confirmed human monkeypox virus cases in Spain: a prospective observational cohort study. Lancet 2022;400(10353):661–9.
45. McLean J, Stoeckle K, Huang S, et al. Tecovirimat Treatment of People With HIV During the 2022 Mpox Outbreak : A Retrospective Cohort Study. Ann Intern Med 2023;176(5):642–8.
46. Fink DL, Callaby H, Luintel A, et al. Clinical features and management of individuals admitted to hospital with monkeypox and associated complications across the UK: a retrospective cohort study. Lancet Infect Dis 2023;23(5):589–97.
47. Abdelaal A, Serhan HA, Mahmoud MA, et al. Ophthalmic manifestations of monkeypox virus. Eye (Lond) 2023;37(3):383–5.
48. Benatti SV, Venturelli S, Comi N, et al. Ophthalmic manifestation of monkeypox infection. Lancet Infect Dis 2022;22(9):1397.
49. Cash Goldwasser SL, Sarah M, McCormick David W, et al. Ocular Monkeypox—United States, July-September 2022. MMWR (Morb Mortal Wkly Rep) 2022; 71(42):1343–7.
50. Adler H, Gould S, Hine P, et al. Clinical features and management of human monkeypox: a retrospective observational study in the UK. Lancet Infect Dis 2022; 22(8):1153–62.
51. Lim CK, McKenzie C, Deerain J, et al. Correlation between monkeypox viral load and infectious virus in clinical specimens. J Clin Virol 2023;161:105421.
52. Nea Matic. Mpox viral load by specimen type and diagnostic testing in a clinical laboratory. Washington: Seattle; 2023. Abstract presented at: CROI; February 19-22.
53. Isolation and Prevention Practices for People with Mpox. Centers for Disease Control and Prevention, National Center for Emerging and Zoonotic Infectious Diseases (NCEZID), Division of High-Consequence Pathogens and Pathology (DHCPP). Updated February 2, 2023. Accessed 6/3/23, https://www.cdc.gov/poxvirus/mpox/clinicians/isolation-procedures.html.
54. Riser APHA, Cima M, Cima M, et al. Epidemiologic and clinical features of mpox-associated deaths—United States May 10,2022-March 7, 2023. MMWR (Morb Mortal Wkly Rep) 2023;72:404–10.
55. Prasad S, Galvan Casas C, Strahan AG, et al. A dermatologic assessment of 101 mpox (monkeypox) cases from 13 countries during the 2022 outbreak: Skin lesion morphology, clinical course, and scarring. J Am Acad Dermatol 2023; 88(5):1066–73.

56. Gross E. Update on emerging infections: news from the centers for disease control and prevention. Ann Emerg Med 2003;42(5):660–4.
57. Luong Nguyen LB, Ghosn J, Durier C, et al. A prospective national cohort evaluating ring MVA vaccination as post-exposure prophylaxis for monkeypox. Nat Med 2022;28(10):1983–4.
58. Pittman PR, Hahn M, Lee HS, et al. Phase 3 efficacy trial of modified vaccinia ankara as a vaccine against smallpox. N Engl J Med 2019;381(20):1897–908.
59. Brooks JTM, Peter Goldstein, Robert H, et al. Intradermal vaccination for monkeypox—benefits for individual and public health. N Engl J Med 2022;387(13):1151–3.
60. Deputy NP, Deckert J, Chard AN, et al. Vaccine effectiveness of JYNNEOS against Mpox Disease in the United States. N Engl J Med 2023;388(26):2434–43.
61. Dalton AF, Diallo AO, Chard AN, et al. Estimated Effectiveness of JYNNEOS Vaccine in Preventing Mpox: A Multijurisdictional Case-Control Study - United States, August 19, 2022-March 31, 2023. MMWR Morb Mortal Wkly Rep 2023;72(20):553–8.
62. Rosenberg EDV, HArt-Malloy R, Hart-Malloy R, et al. Effectiveness of JYNNEOS vaccine against diagnosed Mpox infection — New York 2022. MMWR Morb Mortal Wkly Rep 2023;72:559–63.
63. Bertran M, Andrews N, Davison C, et al. Effectiveness of one dose of MVA-BN smallpox vaccine against mpox in England using the case-coverage method: an observational study. Lancet Infect Dis 2023;23(7):828–35.
64. Wolff Sagy Y, Zucker R, Hammerman A, et al. Real-world effectiveness of a single dose of mpox vaccine in males. Nat Med 2023;29(3):748–52.
65. Duffy JMP, Moro P, Moro P, et al. Safety monitoring of JYNNEOS vaccine during the 2022 Mpox Outbreak — United States, May 22–October 21, 2022. MMWR Morb Mortal Wkly Rep 2022;71:1555–9.
66. Frey SEG, Johannes B, Beigel John H. Erythema and induraion after Mpox (JYNNEOS) vaccination revisited. N Engl J Med 2023;388(15):1432–5.
67. Frey SE, Wald A, Edupuganti S, et al. Comparison of lyophilized versus liquid modified vaccinia Ankara (MVA) formulations and subcutaneous versus intradermal routes of administration in healthy vaccinia-naive subjects. Vaccine 2015;33(39):5225–34.
68. Kota KK, Hong J, Zelaya C, et al. Racial and ethnic disparities in Mpox cases and vaccination among adult males - United States, May-December 2022. MMWR Morb Mortal Wkly Rep 2023;72(15):398–403.
69. Whitehouse ER, Bonwitt J, Hughes CM, et al. Clinical and Epidemiological Findings from Enhanced Monkeypox Surveillance in Tshuapa Province, Democratic Republic of the Congo During 2011-2015. J Infect Dis 2021;223(11):1870–8.
70. Raccagni AR, Canetti D, Mileto D, et al. Two individuals with potential monkeypox virus reinfection. Lancet Infect Dis 2023;23(5):522–4.
71. Golden J, Harryman L, Crofts M, et al. Case of apparent mpox reinfection. Sex Transm Infect 2023;99(4):283–4.
72. Prevention CfDCa. Clinical Considerations for Pain Management of Mpox. Updated March 27, 2023. Accessed June 15, 2023. https://www.cdc.gov/poxvirus/mpox/clinicians/pain-management.html.
73. Emergency Response GRC, WHO Headquarters (HQ). Clinical management and infection prevention and control for monkeypox: Interim rapid response guidance, 10 June 2022. 2022. June 10, 2022. https://www.who.int/publications/i/item/WHO-MPX-Clinical-and-IPC-2022.

74. Grosenbach DW, Honeychurch K, Rose EA, et al. Oral Tecovirimat for the Treatment of Smallpox. N Engl J Med 2018;379(1):44–53.
75. Prevention CfDCa. Information for Healthcare Providers: Tecovirimat (TPOXX) for Treatment of Mpox. Accessed June 15, 2023. https://www.cdc.gov/poxvirus/mpox/clinicians/obtaining-tecovirimat.html#Tecovirimat-IND-Protocol.
76. Prevention CfDCa. Demographics of Patients Receiving TPOXX for Treatment of Mpox. Accessed June 15, 2023. https://www.cdc.gov/poxvirus/mpox/response/2022/demographics-TPOXX.html.
77. O'Laughlin K, Tobolowsky FA, Elmor R, et al. Clinical Use of Tecovirimat (Tpoxx) for Treatment of Monkeypox Under an Investigational New Drug Protocol - United States, May-August 2022. MMWR Morb Mortal Wkly Rep 2022;71(37):1190–5.
78. Mazzotta V, Cozzi-Lepri A, Lanini S, et al. Effect of tecovirimat on healing time and viral clearance by emulation of a target trial in patients hospitalized for mpox. J Med Virol 2023;95(6):e28868.
79. Raccagni AR, Candela C, Bruzzesi E, et al. Real-life use of cidofovir for the treatment of severe monkeypox cases. J Med Virol 2023;95(1):e28218.
80. Stafford A, Rimmer S, Gilchrist M, et al. Use of cidofovir in a patient with severe mpox and uncontrolled HIV infection. Lancet Infect Dis 2023;23(6):e218–26.
81. Quenelle DC, Prichard MN, Keith KA, et al. Synergistic efficacy of the combination of ST-246 with CMX001 against orthopoxviruses. Antimicrob Agents Chemother 2007;51(11):4118–24.
82. Thet AK, Kelly PJ, Kasule SN, et al. The use of Vaccinia Immune Globulin in the Treatment of Severe Mpox. Virus Infection in Human Immunodeficiency Virus/AIDS. Clin Infect Dis 2023;76(9):1671–3.
83. Hyndiuk RA, Seideman S, Leibsohn JM. Treatment of Vaccinial keratitis with trifluorothymidine. Arch Ophthalmol 1976;94(10):1785–6.
84. Pepose JS, Margolis TP, LaRussa P, et al. Ocular complications of smallpox vaccination. Am J Ophthalmol 2003;136(2):343–52.
85. Perzia B, Theotoka D, Li K, et al. Treatment of ocular-involving monkeypox virus with topical trifluridine and oral tecovirimat in the 2022 monkeypox virus outbreak. Am J Ophthalmol Case Rep 2023;29:101779.
86. Prevention CfDCa. Risk Assessment of Mpox Resurgence and Vaccination Considerations. Updated April 4, 2023. Accessed June 10, 2023. https://www.cdc.gov/poxvirus/mpox/response/2022/risk-assessment-of-resurgence.html.

Recurrent Infectious Vaginitis

A Practical Approach for the Primary Care Clinician

Golsa M. Yazdy, MD[a], Caroline Mitchell, MD, MPH[b], Jack D. Sobel, MD[c], Susan Tuddenham, MD, MPH[d,*]

KEYWORDS

- Recurrent vaginitis • Recurrent vulvovaginal candidiasis
- Recurrent bacterial vaginosis • Vulvovaginal candidiasis • Bacterial vaginosis
- Vulvar symptoms

KEY POINTS

- The most common causes of recurrent infectious vaginitis in reproductive-aged individuals are bacterial vaginosis (BV) and vulvovaginal candidiasis (VVC), though other infectious and noninfectious etiologies are possible and should be considered in patients with recurrent symptoms.
- A detailed history and physical examination with appropriate testing at the time of symptoms is critical to establishing a correct diagnosis.
- Recurrent BV and recurrent VVC are defined by three or more confirmed symptomatic episodes in 1 year. Treatment options are limited.
- Complex cases including those with atypical symptoms, negative testing for common causes, refractory symptoms despite appropriate therapy or recurrences during suppressive therapy will require referral to specialist care.

INTRODUCTION

Vaginitis, characterized by vulvovaginal itching, irritation, burning, abnormal vaginal discharge, and/or odor, is one of the most common reasons for visits to both primary

[a] Department of Gynecology & Obstetrics, Johns Hopkins University, 4940 Eastern Avenue, Baltimore, MD 21224, USA; [b] Department of Obstetrics and Gynecology, Harvard Medical School, 55 Fruit Street, Boston, MA 02114, USA; [c] Department of Medicine, Division of Infectious Diseases, Wayne State University, 3901 Chrysler Drive Suite 4A, Detroit, MI 48201, USA; [d] Department of Medicine, Division of Infectious Diseases, Johns Hopkins University, 5200 Eastern Avenue, MFL Center Tower, Suite 381, Baltimore, MD 21224, USA

* Corresponding author. Johns Hopkins University, 5200 Eastern Avenue, MFL Center Tower, Suite 381, Baltimore, MD 21224.

E-mail address: studden1@jhmi.edu

Med Clin N Am 108 (2024) 373–392
https://doi.org/10.1016/j.mcna.2023.08.017

care and gynecologic clinics.[1–3] Recurrent vaginitis (ie, three or more confirmed symptomatic episodes within 1 year) occurs in a subset of patients and can lead to significant morbidity, patient frustration, and health care costs.[4–6] The most common causes of recurrent vaginitis in reproductive-aged women are bacterial vaginosis (BV) and vulvovaginal candidiasis (VVC), although other infectious and noninfectious etiologies are also possible.[2] Here, we provide practical guidance for the primary care clinician on the approach to patients with *recurrent infectious vaginitis*. The authors discuss diagnosis, review common causes (focusing on BV and VVC), and conclude with an approach to management. This review focuses on cisgender nonpregnant adult women; recurrent infectious vaginitis in other populations is important but outside of the scope of this review.

INITIAL APPROACH TO THE PATIENT

Differential Diagnosis

When evaluating patients suspected of having recurrent infectious vaginitis, it is important to keep an open mind because patient self-diagnosis is unreliable and even previous clinician diagnosis could be erroneous.[7–9] Examining the patient at the time of symptoms is critical; clinicians should resist treating patients without examination and rigorous testing to confirm the diagnosis. The most common causes of recurrent infectious vaginitis are BV and VVC. However, sexually transmitted infections (STIs) also need to be ruled out. *Trichomonas vaginalis* (TV) is another leading cause of infectious vaginitis. Gonorrhea (NG) and chlamydia (CT) are not specifically associated with vaginitis but may cause cervicitis, which can result in vaginal discharge.[10] Atrophic vaginitis is an important cause of vaginal symptoms in postmenopausal and breastfeeding women which is sometimes misdiagnosed as BV or VVC. Other less common causes of vaginitis symptoms are possible, and patients suspected of having these entities will need specialist referral (**Table 1**, for some possible causes).[2]

Taking a Patient History

A thorough medical history should be obtained to assess a broad differential diagnosis, including noninfectious causes or environmental exposures (**Table 2**).[1,2,11] Specific symptomatology should be queried (vaginal discharge [color, consistency, amount], irritation, itch, odor, dysuria, dyspareunia), with careful attention to timing, location, duration, and inciting factors or triggers. Although patterns of symptoms may help inform the differential, symptoms alone are not predictive of diagnosis.[1] It is important to educate patients that although vaginal discharge can be pathologic, some degree of vaginal discharge is expected and physiologic.[2] Localized itching, particularly if associated with a focal examination finding, could raise concern for possible vulvar intraepithelial neoplasia or malignancy. Reviewing personal care practices is important use of certain soaps or detergents, hair removal products, menstrual pads, pantiliner, lubricants, or moisturizers can be associated with irritant dermatitis. Patients should be advised against douching or cleaning inside the vagina.[2,11]

Physical Examination and Initial Testing

A physical examination with pelvic evaluation is recommended for all patients presenting with symptoms of recurrent infectious vaginitis. Examination should ideally be performed in symptomatic patients without current vaginal bleeding, who have not recently used vaginal products. A complete examination includes evaluation of the

Table 1
Causes of recurrent vaginitis symptoms

	Symptoms (While Common Symptoms Are Listed, These Are Not Comprehensive; Please Note Symptoms Alone Are Insufficient for Diagnosis)	Examination-Possible Findings	Microscopy-Possible Findings
Common			
Vulvovaginal candidiasis	• Cardinal symptoms: itching and irritation (if absent, symptomatic VVC less likely) • Burning, thick/white discharge, dyspareunia, dysuria	• Erythema of labia majora, minora, and/or vestibule. • Vulvar fissures, excoriations, and/or edema. • Vaginal erythema • White inhomogeneous vaginal discharge • Some patients will have no clear examination findings	Pseudohyphae or budding yeast (though sensitivity is poor).
Bacterial vaginosis	• Cardinal symptoms: increased vaginal discharge and odor (sometimes worse with intercourse)	• No common vulvar findings • Thin, homogenous grayish-white vaginal discharge, elevated pH (>4.5), "fishy" odor on KOH "whiff" test	Clue cells (>20%), absent inflammation (generally no increases in WBC)
Common in postmenopausal individuals			
Vulvovaginal atrophy/atrophic vaginitis	• Vaginal dryness, burning, pain, itching, irritation, urinary symptoms	• May see: decreased volume of labia majora, atrophy of labia minora, architectural changes, pallor of vestibule • Vaginal inflammation and hyperemia, pallor, dryness, loss of rugae • Yellowish discharge, elevated pH (often >5.0)	Parabasal cells present. Normal or increased inflammation (increased WBC)

(*continued on next page*)

Table 1
(*continued*)

	Symptoms (While Common Symptoms Are Listed, These Are Not Comprehensive; Please Note Symptoms Alone Are Insufficient for Diagnosis)	Examination-Possible Findings	Microscopy-Possible Findings
Less common alternative infectious causes of recurrent vaginitis symptoms			
Trichomonas vaginalis	• Most are asymptomatic • Symptomatic: vaginal odor, discharge, itching, dysuria, dyspareunia	• No common vulvar findings • May see: frothy/malodorous/ yellow-green vaginal discharge often with elevated pH (>4.5) • Rarely, colpitis macularis ("strawberry cervix")	Motile trichomonads (though sensitivity is poor). Moderate to severe inflammation (increased WBC)
Cervicitis/pelvic inflammatory disease (PID)	• Many are asymptomatic • Symptomatic: abnormal vaginal discharge, intermenstrual or postcoital bleeding, those with PID may complain of abdominal/pelvic pain	• Cervicitis: purulent or mucopurulent exudate at the endocervix and/or cervical friability (bleeding with gentle touch of cotton swab through cervical os) • PID: cervical, adnexal, or uterine tenderness on bimanual examination • Should be tested for NG/CT/TV, MG testing may be considered if recurrent/refractory. • Should be screened for syphilis and HIV	May see leukorrhea (>10 WBC per hpf)
Herpes simplex virus (HSV)	• Classically painful genital ulcers, dysuria. • However may present with itching/ irritative symptom, mild tingling. Many asymptomatic.	• Classically: vesicular or ulcerative lesions • However, less typical presentations, eg, fissures are also reported. Recurrent unilateral symptoms may occur.	No specific findings

Uncommon causes of recurrent vaginitis symptoms-require specialist referral[a]			
Group A Streptococcus vaginitis	• Discharge, discomfort, itching, dysuria, pain, and/or bleeding	• No common vulvar findings • Discharge (sometimes copious, green or yellow, blood-streaked)	Moderate to severe inflammation (WBC), parabasal cells may be present
Desquamative inflammatory vaginitis	• Symptomatic: stinging, burning, dyspareunia, tenderness, heavy discharge (can be yellow or green) • Long-lasting symptoms that fluctuate in intensity	• No common vulvar findings, vestibule may have petechiae • Vaginal and cervical erythema and petechiae • Purulent discharge (sometimes copious, green or yellow, blood-streaked) with elevated pH (>4.5) and negative whiff test	Moderate to severe inflammation (WBC), parabasal cells present
Vulvar dermatoses (lichen sclerosus, lichen simplex chronicus, lichen planus)	• Itching, pain, burning, soreness, superficial exudate, dyspareunia	• Vulvar skin changes varying from color change, change in skin texture, possible architectural changes, and erosions • Lichen planus can involve the vagina, causing painful erosions, especially at the introitus, and causing agglutination and vaginal adhesions	Lichen planus may have moderate to severe inflammation (WBC) with parabasal cells present.
Irritant dermatitis, eczema	• Itching, pain, superficial exudate	• Ranges from mild erythema and swelling to marked erythema, excoriations, erosions, ulcers	No characteristic findings (no vaginal involvement)
Vulvar intraepithelial lesion/ malignancy	• Itching, pain	• Often visible, raised lesion (but can be flat) • Color can vary (white, gray, red, brown, black, ulcerated)	No characteristic findings (generally no vaginal involvement)
Vulvodynia/vestibulodynia	• Pain or burning at vulva or vulvar vestibule • Multiple possible etiologies (infectious, inflammatory, hormonal, neuropathic)	• Pain with Q-tip test at vulva or vulvar vestibule	Varies by etiology
High-tone pelvic floor dysfunction	• Burning, irritation, pain, dyspareunia, urinary frequency/ urgency/dysuria	• Tenderness and/or increased tension in pelvic floor	No characteristic findings

Abbreviations: CT, chlamydia; hpf, high powered field; KOH, potassium hydroxide; MG, *Mycoplasma genitalium*; NG, gonorrhea; TV, *Trichomonas vaginalis*; WBC, white blood cells.

[a] Not comprehensive—there may be other rare etiologies.

Table 2
Key features of the patient history

History	Key Characteristics	Notes
Symptoms	Refractory vs recurrent symptoms	Refractory—ie, symptoms with no significant improvement after treatment. Refractory symptoms increase concern for drug resistance (eg, in VVC or rarely in TV) or an alternative cause.
	VVC: itching, irritation, discharge *BV*: odor, discharge *TV*: may be asymptomatic, irritation, dysuria, itching, discharge, odor	• Mixed infections may occur, but symptoms not classically consistent with the diagnosis raise concern for mis/alternative diagnosis. However, symptoms alone are insufficient for diagnosis • Atypical symptoms (eg, vulvar pain, discharge alone, ulcers) also raise concern for mis/alternative diagnosis. • There may be causes for itching other than VVC (eg, contact dermatitis, lichen sclerosus, lichen simplex chronicus, malignancy).
	Location/timing of symptoms	• Localized itching raises concern for a focal abnormality (eg, vulvar intraepithelial neoplasia, malignancy). • Perianal itching raises concern for pinworms.
History of prior vaginitis episodes	Initial associated factors (eg, new sexual partner, medications, behaviors). How were they diagnosed	• New or multiple sexual partners raises concern for possible STI • Previous diagnosis and treatment may have been based on symptoms—not verified by full examination or testing. • Review documentation for full Amsel's criteria, microscopy, molecular testing, or fungal culture (in the case of VVC), and PCR-based STI testing. If not performed, diagnosis may be in question.
	Relation of symptoms to menstrual cycle	• Menses may be a trigger for some with BV. • Symptoms may remit during menses for some with VVC. • Symptoms associated temporally with menses could also indicate sensitivity/allergic reaction to menstrual hygiene products.

	Triggers (menses, medications, sex)	• Sex and menses a common trigger for BV, antibiotics a common trigger for VVC.
	Treatment response to clinician prescribed therapies	• Refractory symptoms or symptoms despite what should be effective suppressive therapy raise questions about drug resistance (in VVC) or wrong diagnosis.
	Self-treatment (OTC, alternative or herbal preparations, intravaginal boric acid)	• Can obscure examination or be associated with allergic reaction/sensitivity.
Personal care practices	Hair removal, soaps, pads/pantiliners, lubricants/moisturizers, washing inside the vagina, douching	• Personal care and menstrual practices could be associated with allergic reaction/sensitivity.
Sexual history	# partners, new partners, partners with known STIs, condom use, last STI/HIV testing, dyspareunia, anatomic sexual exposure sites.	• Important to identify need for STI screening or testing. • Female partners with BV symptoms—patient and partner should be assessed and treated as indicated. • Latex condoms and semen are rare potential irritants. • Dryness may cause dyspareunia and mechanical irritation with intercourse; this is common with atrophic changes (postpartum, peri-/postmenopause). • High-tone pelvic floor dysfunction may cause dyspareunia, vulvar itching/burning.
Other medical history/family history	Menopause status, skin conditions, auto-immune conditions, immunocompromising conditions including HIV, diabetes, pregnancy status, smoking	• Vaginitis symptoms could relate to genitourinary syndrome of menopause. • Various skin conditions could manifest as vaginitis symptoms. • Patients with immunocompromise may be at increased risk of VVC. • This review does not focus on pregnancy, but some vaginitis symptoms may be common in pregnancy; pregnancy also affects which medications can be used for treatment. • Recurrent VVC can run in families.
Medications	Use of hormonal contraception, intravaginal estrogen, other medications, OTC, or herbal remedies (eg, intravaginal boric acid)	• Prolonged use of combined oral contraceptive pills (estrogen/progesterone) can be associated with pain/irritation (vestibulodynia). • Vaginal estrogen use has been associated with VVC. • Certain medications may be associated with symptoms (eg, rarely rituximab with inflammatory vaginitis) or predispose to vaginitis.

Abbreviations: BV, bacterial vaginosis; OTC, over the counter; STI, sexually transmitted infection; VVC, vulvovaginal candidiasis.

vulva and perineum for masses, lesions or skin findings, followed by speculum examination to assess for cervicovaginal inflammation, discharge or lesions, and finally a bimanual examination with evaluation for cervical, uterine, and adnexal tenderness. Tenderness at the vaginal introitus should be noted, as this may indicate a noninfectious etiology such as vulvodynia. Bimanual examination should always be done in patients with evidence of cervicitis on examination or complaints of pelvic pain to assess for pelvic inflammatory disease (PID) (**Table 3**).[2,10]

In those with recurrent vaginitis, testing for infectious causes should be comprehensive. Sensitive tests for NG, CT, and TV (ie, polymerase chain reaction [PCR]-based) should be conducted if not already performed. In symptomatic patients in whom recurrent VVC (rVVC) (≥3 episodes in a year) is suspected, a vaginal fungal culture is essential; if this is not available, at least PCR-based testing for *Candida* species should be performed. Antifungal susceptibility testing should be done in women with proven rVVC in whom drug resistance is suspected (ie, when VVC persists and fails to respond to antifungal therapy in treatment-adherent individuals or following breakthrough VVC symptoms while receiving suppressive therapy). BV should be assessed by examination and measurement of vaginal pH, whiff test, and saline microscopy or by a molecular assay that targets more than one BV-associated bacterial species, as recurrent positive tests which only identify *Gardnerella vaginalis* may not represent BV. Microscopy allows assessment of white blood cells (WBC) in the vaginal fluid, which might indicate other causes of symptoms (see **Table 3**, for physical examination findings; **Table 1**, for common microscopy findings; and **Table 4**, for recommended initial testing).[2,3,10,12]

Routine testing for *Ureaplasma parvum, Ureaplasma urealyticum,* and *Mycoplasma hominis* is not recommended as they may be colonizers and are not recognized currently as vaginal pathogens.[13] Testing for *Mycoplasma genitalium* (MG) in the setting of vaginitis symptoms alone is not guideline recommended, though may be considered in individuals with recurrent or refractory cervicitis or PID.[10] Routine genital cultures or molecular tests, including for group B streptococcus, are not recommended.

RECURRENT BACTERIAL VAGINOSIS AND VULVOVAGINAL CANDIDIASIS: THE MOST COMMON CAUSES OF RECURRENT INFECTIOUS VAGINITIS

Recurrent Bacterial Vaginosis

Epidemiology/pathophysiology

BV represents the most common cause of vaginitis symptoms in women of reproductive age[1] and is frequently recurrent—up to 60% of patients recur by 6 months after antibiotic treatment.[14] BV is characterized by a pattern of high-diversity bacterial communities colonizing the vagina ("vaginal microbiota"). A vaginal microbiota characterized by a predominance of *Lactobacillus spp* is associated with optimal reproductive health outcomes, whereas in BV, it becomes dominated by a variety of primarily anaerobic bacteria.[15] Why the condition develops and why it recurs are as yet unresolved. BV is uncommon in women reporting no sexual activity; sexual intercourse as well as menses are commonly reported symptom triggers.[15,16] In epidemiologic studies, an increased number of male sexual partners or having a female partner with a concurrent BV diagnosis[15,16] are associated with incident and recurrent BV (rBV), whereas condom use and male partner circumcision[16] are associated with decreased incident BV. The use of hormonal contraception (HC), in particular estrogen-containing compounds,[17] may be protective against BV. Hypotheses for why BV recurs center on whether these recurrences are due to relapse versus

Table 3
Pelvic exam elements

Examination Site	Conducting the Examination	Notes
Vulva[2,60]	Inspect genitocrural folds, mons pubis, bilateral labia majora and minora, clitoris and clitoral hood, vulvar vestibule, perineal body, and perianal region Note changes in color or architecture, erythema, edema, excoriations, fissures, or ulcerations	• Patients with BV generally do not have vulvar findings. • Patients with VVC may have erythema, edema, and/or excoriations. • Other infectious etiologies, for example, herpes simplex virus may have characteristic lesions. • Noninfectious etiologies may also have vulvar findings, for example, vulvar atrophy (architectural changes), vulvar dermatoses (architectural/color changes, erythema, erosions), and vulvar intraepithelial neoplasia/malignancy (color/texture changes, ulceration).
Vagina[2,60]	Using a speculum, examine for any lesions, atrophic changes (pallor, loss of rogation), petechiae, or erythema. Quantity, color, and texture of discharge should also be documented.	• Discharge may change throughout the menstrual cycle.
Cervix[2,60]	Using a speculum, examine for lesions/masses or purulent discharge, friability	• Purulent discharge or friability diagnose cervicitis.
Bimanual exam[2,60]	Assess for cervical/cervical motion tenderness, uterine, adnexal tenderness	• To assess for PID; should certainly be conducted in patients with evidence of cervicitis on examination or complaints of pelvic pain.
Consider: Q-tip test[12]	Using a moistened swab gently touch external structures (identifying localized vulvar symptoms) and the vulvar vestibule (inside Hart's line), noting the presence of pain out of proportion to pressure (vestibulodynia).	• Vestibulodynia can be caused by infectious, inflammatory, neuropathic, or hormonal etiologies

Abbreviations: BV, bacterial vaginosis; PID, pelvic inflammatory disease; VVC, vulvovaginal candidiasis.

Table 4
Recommended initial testing for patients with recurrent infectious vaginitis

Test	Notes
STI testing: specifically for NG, CT,TV	• Recommended in all patients (at least if not conducted previously, retest as indicated by history and guidelines); all patients with cervicitis or concern for PID on examination should have NG, CT, TV testing. • NAAT tests on vaginal or cervical swabs are recommended as the most sensitive and specific for NG, CT, and TV. NAAT tests on urine are also quite sensitive. • Consider MG testing in patients with recurrent or refractory cervicitis or PID only as per CDC STI treatment guidelines. • Syphilis, HIV, and hepatitis screening as per CDC STI treatment guidelines.
Vaginal pH, "whiff" test with 10% KOH, and microscopy with KOH and saline	• Recommended in all patients • BV can be diagnosed via Amsel's criteria if the patient has $\geq$3 of the following four criteria: that is, thin, homogenous vaginal discharge, vaginal pH > 4.5, clue cells (>20% of epithelial cells), and positive whiff test. • pH may be elevated by sampling cervical fluid, or by blood. • Saline slides are examined under 400x power for clue cells (epithelial cells with finely granulated cytoplasm and indistinct borders), trichomonads, pseudohyphae, budding yeast, parabasal cells (immature epithelial cells), and white blood cells (WBC, marker of inflammation). • Trichomonas may also be diagnosed on saline microscopy; however, sensitivity is poor (44%–68%). • The KOH slide is also examined for pseudohyphae and budding yeast, often more easily seen as epithelial cells are lysed. • VVC can be diagnosed if budding yeast, pseudohyphae or hyphae are visualized on KOH microscopy, however sensitivity is poor (50%–70%).
Vaginal fungal culture or PCR (often available as part of molecular "vaginitis panels")	• Fungal culture, (and if this is not available, PCR) is recommended in symptomatic patients suspected of having recurrent VVC.

(*continued on next page*)

Table 4
(*continued*)

Test	Notes
PCR-based tests for BV (usually part of a "vaginitis panel")	• May be considered if Amsel's criteria cannot be reliably collected in symptomatic patients suspected of having recurrent BV • Tests for a single bacterial species only may be sensitive, but not necessarily specific for BV. Tests which evaluate multiple BV-associated organisms are likely more specific. • Enzyme-based point-of-care tests for BV may also be available.

Abbreviations: CT, chlamydia; NAAT, nucleic acid amplification test; NG, gonorrhea; MG, *Mycoplasma genitalium*; PID, pelvic inflammatory disease; TV, *Trichomonas vaginalis*.

See CDC STI treatment guidelines, Centers for Disease Control Sexually Transmitted Infection Treatment Guidelines (https://www.cdc.gov/std/treatment-guidelines/default.htm).

reinfection. Associations with condomless sexual intercourse suggest that reinfection is important in rBV. Yet, large-scale male partner treatment studies have thus far failed to consistently demonstrate reductions in BV recurrence in women.[16] Relapse from incompletely eradicated BV-associated bacteria in the genital tract due to a biofilm, antibiotic sequestration, or antibiotic resistance[18] is another hypothesized mechanism. BV symptoms frequently resolve after treatment but then recur. However, a minority of patients (up to 38%[19] in a study of women with highly recurrent BV) may exhibit symptomatic BV refractory to antibiotic treatment.[18]

Diagnosis

Vaginal odor and discharge are the cardinal symptoms of BV.[1] BV can be clinically diagnosed if at least three out of four Amsel's criteria (ie, thin, homogenous vaginal discharge, vaginal pH > 4.5, clue cells [>20% of epithelial cells], and positive whiff test) are present.[2,20,21] FDA-approved point-of-care vaginal swab-based tests for BV rely on assaying metabolites or enzymes produced by BV-associated bacteria.[22] Increasingly, new molecular tests that detect multiple species of BV-associated bacteria from vaginal swabs are available. Older tests were DNA probes that focused only on detecting *G vaginalis*; however, the specificity of these tests is questionable given that up to 55% of women without BV might harbor *G vaginalis*.[22] Newer generation tests detect multiple species of vaginal bacteria and may be multiplexed with tests that also detect STIs or candida. However, these tests are not generally available as point of care and are significantly more expensive than the traditional Amsel's criteria. Testing should be performed only in symptomatic patients because treatment of asymptomatic BV is not recommended.[10]

Behavioral or non-pharmacologic recommendations for patients with recurrent bacterial vaginosis

Little data support non-pharmacologic measures to prevent BV recurrences. Based on epidemiologic studies suggesting sharing of microbiota between consistent sexual partners, use of condoms with male partners, cleaning of sex toys between uses, and not sharing toys with female partners should be recommended. Clinicians should recommend against vaginal douching (associated with an increased risk of PID)[23] as well as smoking (which may be linked to increased BV risk); however, there is currently no robust data to suggest that cessation of either practice will reduce BV recurrence.[24,25] Although combined estrogen–progestin contraceptives are associated with lower prevalence of BV, there is currently no robust data to support counseling patients to initiate HC as a means to decrease rBV.[17] Given epidemiologic associations[26] and theoretic concerns regarding biofilm formation, removal of copper intrauterine device (IUDs) may be considered.[2] However, to date, there are no trials to demonstrate that removal of IUDs will result in decreases in rBV recurrences.

Finally, patients often ask about taking probiotics for rBV prevention. Although a recent Phase 2b trial of an intravaginal *Lactobacillus crispatus* live biotherapeutic product to prevent BV recurrence showed some modest benefit,[27] this product is not yet commercially available. Although the idea of using *Lactobacillus*-based probiotic products to improve the vaginal microbiota in women with rBV is theoretically attractive, there is insufficient evidence currently to recommend their use. Moreover, currently available probiotics are of uncertain purity and viability, are mainly oral formulations (which may or may not reach the vagina), and generally contain gut-derived lactobacilli rather than the specific species of *Lactobacillus* commonly found in the vagina.

Pharmacologic intervention

First-line antibiotic recommendations for acute BV episodes include metronidazole 500 mg orally 2 times/day for 7 days, or metronidazole gel 0.75% one full applicator (5 g) intravaginally, once a day for 5 days, or clindamycin cream 2% one full applicator (5 g) intravaginally at bedtime for 7 days.[10,28] Most women will experience resolution of BV symptoms after antibiotic treatment, but symptoms may recur soon after. Alternative treatments may include oral clindamycin, secnidazole, tinidazole, or alternative formulations of intravaginal clindamycin or metronidazole, but no single regimen has been shown to have superior efficacy or improved outcomes over first-line therapy.[10,28]

Symptomatic women with rBV should be treated with a multiday first-line regimen. A switch to an alternative first-line recommended drug class may be considered (ie, metronidazole to clindamycin or vice versa), though in studies of those with acute BV overall outcomes for treatment are similar.[10,18] Of note, patients should be counseled that clindamycin intravaginal cream is oil-based and might weaken latex condoms and diaphragms for 5 days after use. In those who continue to have recurrences, guidelines suggest that patients may be prescribed suppressive vaginal metronidazole after acute treatment (0.75% metronidazole vaginal gel one applicatorful twice weekly for 4–6 months).[10,28] While not Food and Drug Administration (FDA) approved for this purpose, this dosing regimen of metronidazole gel is supported by a randomized controlled trial which showed prevention of recurrence in nearly 70% of women while on therapy, though treatment was complicated by VVC in 40%; recurrences were common after therapy was stopped[29] (**Fig. 1**). Alternative regimens have been reported in the literature[30,31] and are cited in guidelines[10] but have not been studied in randomized controlled trials and cannot be routinely recommended. Specialist referral is recommended for patients experiencing recurrent symptoms despite suppressive therapy.

Refractory BV (ie, where symptoms do not remit and the patient still meets criteria for BV despite treatment) is an entity that is only recently being recognized as a clinical issue and is not as yet discussed in national guidelines.[18] Exact incidence is uncertain. In the absence of data, similar to rBV, it may be reasonable to retreat with a multiday regimen, possibly switching route of therapy (eg, vaginal to oral) or consider a switch to an alternative first-line recommended drug class.[18] If patients remain refractory after this therapy specialist referral is advised.

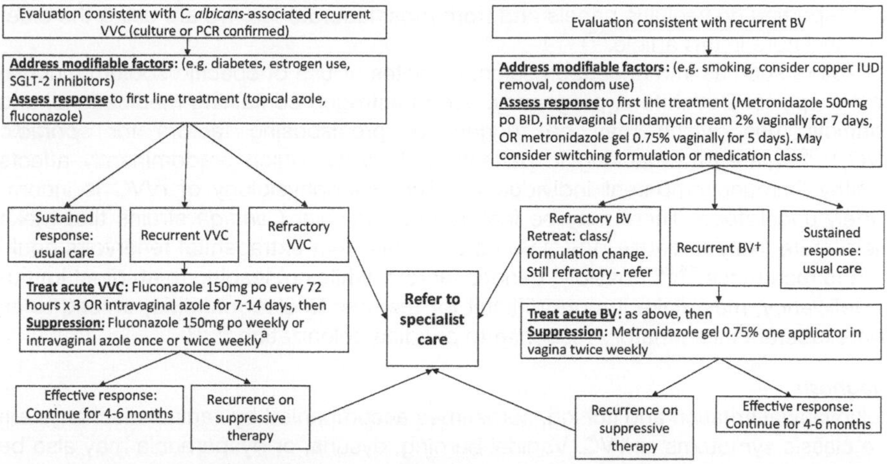

Fig. 1. Initial management of patients with rVVC or rBV. [a]Ibrexafungerp and oteseconazole have also been FDA-approved in specific regimens for rVVC but are not yet included in guidelines. Fluconazole should not be used in pregnancy. [b]See text for discussion of rBV in postmenopausal individuals. BV, bacterial vaginosis; po, orally; VVC, vulvovaginal candidiasis.

At this time, robust data to support treatment of male partners to prevent BV recurrences are lacking, although this continues to be an active area of research. Symptomatic female partners should be evaluated and treated if found to have BV.[10,18]

Postmenopausal patients

Postmenopausal individuals are challenging to manage as they have been excluded from much of BV research and diagnostic methods were not originally studied in this population. The physiologic lowering of systemic estrogen levels in these individuals may alter the vaginal microbiota, decreasing lactobacilli and increasing vaginal pH, confounding the diagnosis. Genital itching, irritation, burning, discharge and sometimes odor may be reported by women experiencing the genitourinary syndrome of menopause. In postmenopausal women with repeated complaints of vaginitis symptoms and no other clear etiology for symptoms, it is reasonable to trial vaginal estrogen therapy or to refer these patients to a gynecologist for consideration of this therapy, particularly if there are signs of atrophy on examination and/or parabasal cells on saline microscopy are noted. Postmenopausal patients meeting Amsel's criteria should be treated for BV, but then similarly could be considered for vaginal estrogen therapy to see if this decreases symptom recurrences.[32]

Recurrent Vulvovaginal Candidiasis

Epidemiology/pathophysiology

VVC, inflammation of the vulva and vagina caused by fungal infection, occurs at least once in 23% to 49% (up to 75% in some estimates) of women.[5,33] Of these, between 14% and 28% may experience rVVC ($\geq$3–4 episodes in a 1-year period).[33] *Candida albicans* is responsible for the majority (80%–95%) of VVC and rVVC. More rarely, other yeast species (most commonly *Candida glabrata*, but also *Candida krusei*, *Candida parapsilosis,* and *Candida tropicalis*) have been reported to cause VVC.[34–36] (Note: nomenclature for *Candida* has recently changed, but for clarity and to be consistent with reporting on vaginitis panels and from most laboratories, we are using the older nomenclature in this article.[37])

Factors such as immunosuppression, diabetes or use of specific sodium glucose co-transporter 2 inhibitors, pregnancy, use of estrogen-containing medications, and antibiotic use, which may be triggers or predisposing factors for *sporadic* VVC,[35,36,38] are often lacking in patients with rVVC, which predominantly affects healthy, immunocompetent individuals.[35] The pathophysiology of rVVC is incompletely understood. There may be features of particular *Candida* strains that make them more likely to cause rVVC. Some speculate that extragenital reservoirs could lead to recurrence.[35,36] Possibly, genetic factors, while not leading to an overt immunodeficiency, may make it more difficult for the host to clear candida, or lead to an overexuberant inflammatory response to candida colonization.[35,36]

Diagnosis

Vulvovaginal irritation and itching, sometimes accompanied by vaginal discharge are the classic symptoms of VVC. Vaginal burning, dysuria, or dyspareunia may also be reported.[10,28] Diagnosis of VVC is ideally made in the context of consistent symptoms with the presence of candida documented on microscopy, a positive nucleic acid amplification testing (NAAT) test or positive vaginal fungal culture. However, microscopy is insensitive for diagnosis of yeast (50%–70%).[10,28] Although unnecessary in sporadic VVC, in patients with rVVC, vaginal fungal culture or PCR is recommended to verify the presence of candida and identify *Candida* species responsible. Asymptomatic vaginal colonization with candida occurs in up to 20% of women and does not necessitate treatment. Thus, *causality*, that is, whether fungi detected in the vagina are truly responsible for symptoms as opposed to only colonizers must always be determined. This issue is particularly relevant for non-albicans *Candida* species which are less virulent and are less likely to be responsible for symptoms.[2,5,28]

Behavioral or non-pharmacologic recommendations for patients with recurrent vulvovaginal candidiasis

If there are modifiable predisposing factors or triggers for VVC, these should be addressed (see **Fig. 1**). Patients also often ask about dietary measures; however, there are little data to support any particular dietary regimen to be avoided or recommended. Probiotics designed "for vaginal health" aim to support the growth of lactobacilli, but available data suggest vaginal candida may actually be more common in women with *Lactobacillus*-dominated vaginal microbiota.[39] Given lack of data, probiotics or dietary measures to prevent VVC cannot be recommended.

Treatment

Guideline-recommended treatment regimens for uncomplicated acute symptomatic VVC include fluconazole 150 mg orally in a single dose and various intravaginal azole regimens with regimens ranging from 1 to 7 days. Severe acute VVC may require slightly longer courses.[10,28] For patients with rVVC, each acute symptomatic episode may be treated individually. However, in patients with greater than 3 symptomatic recurrences in a year, suppressive/prophylactic therapy may be considered. Suppressive therapy is typically initiated after an "induction" treatment course (eg, a topical azole [one applicatorful in vagina daily for 7–14 days] or 3 doses of fluconazole 150 mg, given 72 hours apart[10,28]) followed by weekly therapy for 4 to 6 months.[10,28] The best studied regimen is weekly fluconazole 150 mg.[10,28] Per guidelines, a topical azole (eg, clotrimazole) used once or twice weekly can also be considered if there are concerns about tolerability, medication interactions, or pregnancy.[10,28] Of note, fluconazole has been associated with spontaneous abortion and congenital anomalies and therefore should not be used in pregnancy[10] (see **Fig. 1**). Excellent rates of remission are achieved while on suppressive prophylactic fluconazole therapy, though patients may recur once suppressive therapy is stopped.[40]

Recently two new medications were FDA-approved for treatment of rVVC, ibrexafungerp and oteseconazole. Ibrexafungerp is approved for acute VVC in a 1-day regimen and for rVVC with monthly dosing for 6 months but like fluconazole cannot be used in pregnancy.[41] Oteseconazole has an extraordinarily long half-life of 138 days, is approved only for rVVC, and has a multidose regimen taken for 3 months. It is only recommended for patients with no childbearing potential given its long half-life and potential to cause fetal harm. Ibrexafungerp and oteseconazole use is not yet in guidelines and is expensive.[42]

Azole resistance

Although most of rVVC is thought to be caused by fluconazole sensitive *C. albicans*, fluconazole resistance has been reported. Fluconazole resistance is relatively common in non-albicans species such as *C. glabrata*[43] and is predictable in *C. krusei*. Fluconazole resistance in *C. albicans* has historically been considered to be rare[44]; however, emerging data suggest vaginal *C. albicans* fluconazole resistance may be more common than previously recognized[43,45,46] and may be increasing.[45,47] Fluconazole resistance in *C. albicans* has been associated with clinical treatment failure.[46]

If patients present with recurrent symptoms while on suppressive fluconazole therapy, an alternative diagnosis or antifungal resistance should be considered and patients should be referred to specialist care. Patients with non-albicans *Candida* isolated vaginally who have symptoms consistent with VVC should also be referred for specialist care.

LESS COMMON INFECTIOUS AND NONINFECTIOUS CAUSES OF RECURRENT VAGINITIS SYMPTOMS

Infectious Causes

TV, a sexually transmitted parasite, is highly prevalent, including in women over age 40.[48–52] While asymptomatic in most, TV is an important cause of vaginitis symptoms and can also infect the cervix, urethra, and Skene and Bartholin glands.[49,51,52] TV has been associated with PID, particularly in women with HIV.[53,54] Diagnosis of TV can be made on microscopy of vaginal secretions, but sensitivity is only 44% to 68%; NAAT tests (which can be conducted on vaginal, endocervical, or urine specimens) are the most sensitive and are preferred.[51] Several point-of-care molecular tests for TV are also now available.[51] As a common infectious cause of vaginitis, TV should be considered at least in the initial evaluation of patients with recurrent vaginitis.[10] Patients testing positive who experience recurrent or refractory symptoms after treatment should be retested. However, NAAT tests should not be used before 3 to 4 weeks have passed after treatment completion because of the possibility of false positives secondary to residual nucleic acid.[10] The most likely cause for recurrent or even refractory TV is reinfection from an inadequately treated partner or poor compliance with therapy. In the relatively small group of patients who have symptoms and test positive for TV again after treatment in whom reinfection or poor compliance does not seem to be at issue, resistant TV should be considered. Treatment failures related to nitroimidazole resistance have been reported; however, only 4% to 10% of isolates generally exhibit some level of nitroimidazole resistance.[55–57] In women with persistent TV in whom reinfection or poor compliance has been ruled out, guidelines suggest treatment with metronidazole or tinidazole 2 g once daily for 7 days. However, if patients fail this regimen, specialist referral is indicated and nitroimidazole resistance testing should be sought—this is available at the CDC.[10]

In terms of other infectious causes, *cervicitis* should be ruled out as a cause for vaginal discharge complaints. The etiology can either be infectious (usually due to CT or NG but TV, MG, and herpes simplex virus (HSV) have also been implicated) or non-infectious.[10] HSV can cause recurrent pain, irritative or itching symptoms; if lesions are noted on examination, NAAT should be performed.[10] *Group A streptococcus* (GAS) infectious vaginitis is a rare entity but has been described as a cause of recurrent vaginitis. In comparison to the skin and throat, vaginal colonization of GAS is uncommon and usually asymptomatic. In adult women, GAS vaginitis may present with discharge, discomfort, itching, dysuria, pain, and/or bleeding. If suspected, a vaginal culture is recommended; however, a positive result could reflect either colonization or infection and must be interpreted in the right clinical context[58,59]; specialist referral is recommended.

Noninfectious Causes

Noninfectious etiologies of vulvovaginal symptoms are not the focus of this review, but there are many, for example, vulvar dermatitis/dermatoses, desquamative inflammatory vaginitis, vulvovaginal atrophy/atrophic vaginitis, vulvodynia/vestibulodynia, vulvar intraepithelial neoplasia/malignancy, and pelvic floor dysfunction. Common presentations of these conditions are reviewed in **Table 1**. If these etiologies are suspected based on patient history or physical examination findings, referral to a specialist is recommended for further evaluation and treatment.[2]

DISCUSSION: INITIAL MANAGEMENT OF PATIENTS

STIs found on initial workup should be treated as appropriate. Patients with negative testing for common causes of recurrent vaginitis should be referred for specialist evaluation. In the case of vulvar skin changes, chronic ulcerations, or lesions, referral to a dermatologist or gynecologist for evaluation and possible biopsy is recommended. If there is high suspicion for malignancy, patients should be referred to a gynecologic oncologist.

For patients whose evaluation seems consistent with rVVC due to *C. albicans* or BV, *setting expectations* for patients upfront is important. Unfortunately, currently available therapies are not likely to eradicate infection in most of those with rVVC or rBV. However, these conditions may be managed with suppressive regimens which do require significant commitment from patients to be effective. After addressing any potential modifiable factors, which may predispose to these vaginal conditions, patients with rBV or rVVC who recur after initial therapy may be considered for suppressive regimens (see **Fig. 1**). Those who have continued or recurrent symptoms while on suppressive regimens should be referred for specialist care. Once suppressive regimens are stopped, a significant proportion of patients may experience symptomatic vaginitis recurrence.

SUMMARY

Recurrent infectious vaginitis, most commonly caused in reproductive-aged women by BV and VVC, is a common problem faced by primary care clinicians. A detailed history and physical examination with appropriate testing at the time of symptoms is critical to establishing a correct diagnosis. Limited but effective suppressive options for rBV and VVC exist. Ultimately, better understanding of pathophysiology and improved regimens to treat and prevent common causes of recurrent infectious vaginitis are needed.

CLINICS CARE POINTS

- The most common causes of recurrent infectious vaginitis are bacterial vaginosis (BV) and vulvovaginal candidiasis (VVC), but other infectious and noninfectious causes also exist.
- A detailed history and physical examination with appropriate testing at the time of symptoms is critical to establishing a correct diagnosis.
- Sexually transmitted infections should be ruled out as a cause of recurrent vaginitis symptoms.
- Localized itching, particularly associated with a focal examination finding, could raise concern for possible vulvar intraepithelial neoplasia or malignancy.
- Atrophic vaginitis is a common cause of vaginitis symptoms in postmenopausal women and may improve with topical estrogen therapy.
- Fungal culture or PCR-based testing is advised for all patients with concern for recurrent vulvovaginal candidiasis to confirm diagnosis and establish speciation.
- Suppressive regimens may be attempted for those with recurrent VVC or recurrent BV; however, complex cases including those with atypical symptoms, negative testing for common causes, refractory symptoms despite appropriate therapy, or recurrences during suppressive therapy will require referral to specialist care.

DISCLOSURE

S. Tuddenham has been a consultant for BioFire Diagnostics, Roche Molecular Diagnostics, and Luca Biologics, receives royalties from UPTODATE, and has received speaker honoraria from Roche Molecular Diagnostics and Medscape/WebMD. She participates in research supported by donation of test kits to her academic institution by Hologic, United States. J.D. Sobel has been a consultant to Scynexis Pharmaceuticals and Mycovia Pharmaceuticals and receives royalties from UPTODATE. C. Mitchell has been a consultant for Ferring Pharmaceuticals and Scynexis. She receives research funding from Scynexis, royalties from Up to Date, and grants from the Bill and Melinda Gates Foundation, United States. G.M. Yazdy has no disclosures.

REFERENCES

1. Anderson MR, Klink K, Cohrssen A. Evaluation of vaginal complaints. JAMA 2004;291(11):1368–79.
2. Editors: Viera-Baptista PS, CK; Sobel J. The International Society for the Study of Vulvovaginal Disease Recommendations for the Diagnosis and Treatment of Vaginitis. 2023; https://www.issvd.org/guidelines.
3. Shroff S. Infectious Vaginitis, Cervicitis, and Pelvic Inflammatory Disease. Med Clin North Am 2023;107(2):299–315.
4. Bilardi JE, Walker S, Temple-Smith M, et al. The burden of bacterial vaginosis: women's experience of the physical, emotional, sexual and social impact of living with recurrent bacterial vaginosis. PLoS One 2013;8(9):e74378.
5. Neal CM, Martens MG. Clinical challenges in diagnosis and treatment of recurrent vulvovaginal candidiasis. SAGE Open Med 2022;10. 20503121221115201.
6. Zhu YX, Li T, Fan SR, et al. Health-related quality of life as measured with the Short-Form 36 (SF-36) questionnaire in patients with recurrent vulvovaginal candidiasis. Health Qual Life Outcome 2016;14:65.

7. Ferris DG, Nyirjesy P, Sobel JD, et al. Over-the-counter antifungal drug misuse associated with patient-diagnosed vulvovaginal candidiasis. Obstet Gynecol 2002;99(3):419–25.
8. Hillier SL, Austin M, Macio I, et al. Diagnosis and Treatment of Vaginal Discharge Syndromes in Community Practice Settings. Clin Infect Dis 2021;72(9):1538–43.
9. Ryan-Wenger NA, Neal JL, Jones AS, et al. Accuracy of vaginal symptom self-diagnosis algorithms for deployed military women. Nurs Res 2010;59(1):2–10.
10. Workowski KA, Bachmann LH, Chan PA, et al. Sexually Transmitted Infections Treatment Guidelines, 2021. MMWR Recomm Rep (Morb Mortal Wkly Rep) 2021;70(4):1–187.
11. Reichman O, Margesson LJ, Rasmussen CA, et al. Algorithms for Managing Vulvovaginal Symptoms-a Practical Primer. Curr Infect Dis Rep 2019;21(10):40.
12. Bornstein J; Goldstein AT, Stockdale CK, et al. 2015 ISSVD, ISSWSH, and IPPS Consensus Terminology and Classification of Persistent Vulvar Pain and Vulvodynia. J Sex Med 2016;13(4):607–12.
13. Horner P, Donders G, Cusini M, et al. Should we be testing for urogenital Mycoplasma hominis, Ureaplasma parvum and Ureaplasma urealyticum in men and women? - a position statement from the European STI Guidelines Editorial Board. J Eur Acad Dermatol Venereol 2018;32(11):1845–51.
14. Bradshaw CS, Morton AN, Hocking J, et al. High recurrence rates of bacterial vaginosis over the course of 12 months after oral metronidazole therapy and factors associated with recurrence. J Infect Dis 2006;193(11):1478–86.
15. Tuddenham S, Ravel J, Marrazzo JM. Protection and Risk: Male and Female Genital Microbiota and Sexually Transmitted Infections. J Infect Dis 2021;223(12 Suppl 2):S222–35.
16. Vodstrcil LA, Muzny CA, Plummer EL, et al. Bacterial vaginosis: drivers of recurrence and challenges and opportunities in partner treatment. BMC Med 2021; 19(1):194.
17. Ratten LK, Plummer EL, Bradshaw CS, et al. The Effect of Exogenous Sex Steroids on the Vaginal Microbiota: A Systematic Review. Front Cell Infect Microbiol 2021;11:732423.
18. Muzny CA, Sobel JD. The Role of Antimicrobial Resistance in Refractory and Recurrent Bacterial Vaginosis and Current Recommendations for Treatment. Antibiotics (Basel) 2022;11(4).
19. Sobel JD, Kaur N, Woznicki NA, et al. Prognostic Indicators of Recurrence of Bacterial Vaginosis. J Clin Microbiol 2019;57(5).
20. Eschenbach DA, Hillier S, Critchlow C, et al. Diagnosis and clinical manifestations of bacterial vaginosis. Am J Obstet Gynecol 1988;158(4):819–28.
21. Amsel R, Totten PA, Spiegel CA, et al. Nonspecific vaginitis. Diagnostic criteria and microbial and epidemiologic associations. Am J Med 1983;74(1):14–22.
22. Coleman JS, Gaydos CA. Molecular Diagnosis of Bacterial Vaginosis: an Update. J Clin Microbiol 2018;56(9).
23. Ness RB, Soper DE, Holley RL, et al. Douching and endometritis: results from the PID evaluation and clinical health (PEACH) study. Sex Transm Dis 2001;28(4): 240–5.
24. Brotman RM, Ghanem KG, Klebanoff MA, et al. The effect of vaginal douching cessation on bacterial vaginosis: a pilot study. Am J Obstet Gynecol 2008; 198(6):628, e621-627.
25. Brotman RM, He X, Gajer P, et al. Association between cigarette smoking and the vaginal microbiota: a pilot study. BMC Infect Dis 2014;14:471.

26. Peebles K, Kiweewa FM, Palanee-Phillips T, et al. Elevated Risk of Bacterial Vaginosis Among Users of the Copper Intrauterine Device: A Prospective Longitudinal Cohort Study. Clin Infect Dis 2021;73(3):513–20.
27. Cohen CR, Wierzbicki MR, French AL, et al. Randomized Trial of Lactin-V to Prevent Recurrence of Bacterial Vaginosis. N Engl J Med 2020;382(20):1906–15.
28. Paavonen JA, Brunham RC. Vaginitis in Nonpregnant Patients: ACOG Practice Bulletin Number 215. Obstet Gynecol 2020;135(5):1229–30.
29. Sobel JD, Ferris D, Schwebke J, et al. Suppressive antibacterial therapy with 0.75% metronidazole vaginal gel to prevent recurrent bacterial vaginosis. Am J Obstet Gynecol 2006;194(5):1283–9.
30. Reichman O, Akins R, Sobel JD. Boric acid addition to suppressive antimicrobial therapy for recurrent bacterial vaginosis. Sex Transm Dis 2009;36(11):732–4.
31. Surapaneni S, Akins R, Sobel JD. Recurrent Bacterial Vaginosis: An Unmet Therapeutic Challenge. Experience With a Combination Pharmacotherapy Long-Term Suppressive Regimen. Sex Transm Dis 2021;48(10):761–5.
32. Van Gerwen OMCA. Bacterial Vaginosis in Postmenopausal Women. Curr Infect Dis Rep 2023;25:7–15.
33. Blostein F, Levin-Sparenberg E, Wagner J, et al. Recurrent vulvovaginal candidiasis. Ann Epidemiol 2017;27(9):575–582 e573.
34. Sobel JD. Vulvovaginal candidosis. Lancet 2007;369(9577):1961–71.
35. Willems HME, Ahmed SS, Liu J, et al. Vulvovaginal Candidiasis: A Current Understanding and Burning Questions. J Fungi (Basel) 2020;6(1).
36. Goncalves B, Ferreira C, Alves CT, et al. Vulvovaginal candidiasis: Epidemiology, microbiology and risk factors. Crit Rev Microbiol 2016;42(6):905–27.
37. Kidd SE, Abdolrasouli A, Hagen F. Fungal Nomenclature: Managing Change is the Name of the Game. Open Forum Infect Dis 2023;10(1):ofac559.
38. Nyirjesy P, Sobel JD, Fung A, et al. Genital mycotic infections with canagliflozin, a sodium glucose co-transporter 2 inhibitor, in patients with type 2 diabetes mellitus: a pooled analysis of clinical studies. Curr Med Res Opin 2014;30(6):1109–19.
39. Brown SE, Schwartz JA, Robinson CK, et al. The Vaginal Microbiota and Behavioral Factors Associated With Genital *Candida albicans* Detection in Reproductive-Age Women. Sex Transm Dis 2019;46(11):753–8.
40. Collins LM, Moore R, Sobel JD. Prognosis and Long-Term Outcome of Women With Idiopathic Recurrent Vulvovaginal Candidiasis Caused by *Candida albicans*. J Low Genit Tract Dis 2020;24(1):48–52.
41. Phillips NA, Rocktashel M, Merjanian L. Ibrexafungerp for the Treatment of Vulvovaginal Candidiasis: Design, Development and Place in Therapy. Drug Des Dev Ther 2023;17:363–7.
42. Sobel JD. New Antifungals for Vulvovaginal Candidiasis: What Is Their Role? Clin Infect Dis 2023;76(5):783–5.
43. Sobel JD, Sobel R. Current treatment options for vulvovaginal candidiasis caused by azole-resistant Candida species. Expet Opin Pharmacother 2018;19(9):971–7.
44. Pappas PG, Kauffman CA, Andes DR, et al. Clinical Practice Guideline for the Management of Candidiasis: 2016 Update by the Infectious Diseases Society of America. Clin Infect Dis 2016;62(4):e1–50.
45. Agrawal P, Yazdy G, Ghanem KG, et al. Vaginal *Candida albicans*: High Frequency of in Vitro Fluconazole Resistance in a Select Population-A Brief Note. Sex Transm Dis 2023;50(2):121–3.
46. File B, Sobel R, Becker M, et al. Fluconazole-Resistant *Candida albicans* Vaginal Infections at a Referral Center and Treated With Boric Acid. J Low Genit Tract Dis 2023.

47. Sobel JD. Resistance to Fluconazole of *Candida albicans* in Vaginal Isolates: a 10-Year Study in a Clinical Referral Center. Antimicrob Agents Chemother 2023;e0018123.
48. Patel EU, Gaydos CA, Packman ZR, et al. Prevalence and Correlates of *Trichomonas vaginalis* Infection Among Men and Women in the United States. Clin Infect Dis 2018;67(2):211–7.
49. Van Gerwen OT, Muzny CA. Recent advances in the epidemiology, diagnosis, and management of *Trichomonas vaginalis* infection. F1000Res 2019;8.
50. Lindrose AR, Htet KZ, O'Connell S, et al. Burden of trichomoniasis among older adults in the United States: a systematic review. Sex Health 2022;19(3):151–6.
51. Van Gerwen OT, Opsteen SA, Graves KJ, et al. Trichomoniasis. Infect Dis Clin North Am 2023;37(2):245–65.
52. Tuddenham S, Hamill MM, Ghanem KG. Diagnosis and Treatment of Sexually Transmitted Infections: A Review. JAMA 2022;327(2):161–72.
53. Moodley P, Wilkinson D, Connolly C, et al. *Trichomonas vaginalis* is associated with pelvic inflammatory disease in women infected with human immunodeficiency virus. Clin Infect Dis 2002;34(4):519–22.
54. Mitchell CM, Anyalechi GE, Cohen CR, et al. Etiology and Diagnosis of Pelvic Inflammatory Disease: Looking Beyond Gonorrhea and Chlamydia. J Infect Dis 2021;224(12 Suppl 2):S29–35.
55. Augostini P, Bradley ELP, Raphael BH, et al. In vitro testing of *Trichomonas vaginalis* drug susceptibility: evaluation of minimal lethal concentrations for metronidazole and tinidazole that correspond with treatment failure. Sex Transm Dis 2023. https://doi.org/10.1097/OLQ.0000000000001788.
56. Secor WE, Meites E, Starr MC, et al. Neglected parasitic infections in the United States: trichomoniasis. Am J Trop Med Hyg 2014;90(5):800–4.
57. Schwebke JR, Barrientes FJ. Prevalence of *Trichomonas vaginalis* isolates with resistance to metronidazole and tinidazole. Antimicrob Agents Chemother 2006;50(12):4209–10.
58. Donders G, Greenhouse P, Donders F, et al. Genital Tract GAS Infection ISIDOG Guidelines. J Clin Med 2021;10(9).
59. Sobel JD, Funaro D, Kaplan EL. Recurrent group A streptococcal vulvovaginitis in adult women: family epidemiology. Clin Infect Dis 2007;44(5):e43–5.
60. Workowski KA, Bachmann LH. Centers for Disease Control and Prevention's Sexually Transmitted Diseases Infection Guidelines. Clin Infect Dis 2022;74(74 Suppl 2):S89–94.

Sexual Health Care for Transgender and Gender Diverse People

Kevin L. Ard, MD, MPH[a,b,*], Andrew MacDonald-Ly, PharmD, AAHIVP[c], A.C Demidont, MD[d]

KEYWORDS

- Transgender • Gender diverse • Sexual health care • Gender-affirming care
- Sexually transmitted infections • HIV

KEY POINTS

- Transgender and gender diverse (TGD) people are those whose gender identities do not align with societal expectations based on their sex assigned at birth. TGD people have faced discrimination within health care and society more broadly which impacts their health, including sexual health.
- Sexual health care for TGD people should be embedded within a gender-affirming context. Strategies to make health care environments more inclusive of TGD people include training all staff about TGD concepts, asking all patients about their names and pronouns, and developing clinical expertise in gender-affirming care.
- To optimize sexual health care for TGD people, clinicians should adopt a mindset of cultural humility, intentionally incorporating shared language norms (mirroring) when describing genital anatomy; approach all health discussions in a trauma-informed manner with special attention to the significant trauma often experienced by TGD patients when discussing secondary sex characteristics and external genitalia; elicit sexual histories that are inclusive of all gender identities; adopt an anatomy-based approach to sexually transmitted infection screening; offer self-collection for gonorrhea and chlamydia testing; and colocate sexual health and gender-affirming services.

INTRODUCTION

Sexual health is an integral part of overall health, and addressing sexual health—including sexual function, satisfaction, and disease—is a core aspect of primary care. As the number of people who identify as transgender or gender diverse (TGD) grows,[1] primary care clinicians will increasingly be called on to provide sexual health

[a] Harvard Medical School; [b] Division of Infectious Diseases, Massachusetts General Hospital, 55 Fruit Street, Boston, MA 02114, USA; [c] Gilead Sciences, Inc, HIV Global Medical Affairs, 333 Lakeside Drive, Foster City, CA 94404, USA; [d] Gilead Sciences, Inc, HIV Treatment Medical Affairs, 333 Lakeside Drive, Foster City, CA 94404, USA
* Corresponding author.
E-mail address: Kard@mgh.harvard.edu

Med Clin N Am 108 (2024) 393–402
https://doi.org/10.1016/j.mcna.2023.10.002

care for TGD patients. Sexual health care for TGD people is similar to sexual health care for cisgender people; the medical and psychosocial sexual history should be sex positive, free of judgment, lacking in assumptions, and cognizant of the potential for low provider and patient sexual health literacy. In addition, clinicians must vigilantly maintain privacy and ensure quality outcomes. Because optimal sexual care for TGD people also requires an understanding of gender identity and expression, creation of care environments that are welcoming to and affirming of TGD people, fluency in sexual health terminology which is applicable and acceptable, knowledge about the impacts of gender-affirming medical care on sexual function and satisfaction, inclusion of voices with lived experience, and/or providers with clinical backgrounds working with TGD patients should inform most, if not all, aspects of care. Involving community members early in the development of clinical services can identify existing care gaps and tactics to close those gaps as well as critical success and performance metrics. In addition, by considering how prior experiences of trauma and discrimination may impact sexual health care for TGD people, clinicians can deliver care that is maximally accessible for these populations.

APPROACH

Here, the authors outline fundamental concepts and approaches to the care of TGD people. The authors then describe how to incorporate these into concrete aspects of sexual health care.

Key Concepts

TGD people are those whose gender identities—their internal sense of being men, women, some of both, or another gender—do not align with societal expectations for their sex assigned at birth. In comparison, people who are cisgender are those whose gender identities align with societal expectations for their sex assigned at birth.[2] The term gender diverse encompasses a range of identities, including people with gender identities that are not binary (nonbinary/genderqueer) or who do not identify with the construct of gender as binary (agender/neutrois). Nonbinary people may or may not consider themselves transgender. Nonbinary gender identities are common; of nearly 28,000 respondents to the 2015 US Transgender Survey, approximately 35% identified as nonbinary, compared with 33% who identified as transgender women and 29% who identified as transgender men.[3] Gender identity is distinct from sexual orientation, which refers to people's romantic or sexual attraction and behavior vis-a-vis others. Like cisgender people, TGD people may have any sexual orientation, and their sexual orientation and behavior may change over time.

For many TGD people, the process of gender affirmation is central to their personal development, clinical care, and survival. Gender affirmation, sometimes called transition, is the process by which people make social, legal, and secondary sex characteristic changes to align physical attributes with their gender identity.[2] These changes may include telling one's friends or family about one's gender identity, changing the gender marker on one's driver's license, and/or taking hormones or undergoing surgeries. Importantly, the process of gender affirmation is unique to each TGD person; there is no correct sequence or order, and people may engage with some aspects of gender affirmation (eg, social affirmation) and not others (eg, surgery). Because of the individual nature of gender affirmation, making assumptions about someone's names and pronouns, hormonal milieu, or anatomy based on their appearance or the sex assigned at birth is prone to error; clinicians should ask this information instead, if needed for medical care.

Cultivating Affirming Care Environments

The most crucial step clinicians can take to foster the health and wellness of TGD people is to create clinical environments that are thoroughly and explicitly inclusive and welcoming. *Thoroughly* means that all aspects of care—from the check-in process at the front desk to the questions clinicians ask in the examination room to the physical environment of the clinic—include and affirm TGD people. **Table 1** highlights strategies to cultivate gender-affirming care environments. Many of these strategies (eg, asking how patients would like to be addressed, providing single stall restrooms) may also improve the experience of cisgender patients.

When approaching care for TGD people, it is helpful to consider the histories of discrimination, exclusion, stigma, and trauma that have shaped the lives of many individuals within these populations and to design care delivery with these considerations in mind. Many TGD people have experienced violence and anti-transgender acts of discrimination, including within health care settings.[3] For example, one-third of TGD people report negative experiences with clinicians, including being harassed or denied care because of their gender identities, frequently leading them to avoid or delay seeking medical attention when it was needed.[3] By taking steps to make clinical settings more welcoming for TGD people and providing care for all people through

Table 1
Strategies and examples to foster gender-affirming clinical environments

Strategy	Example
Train staff about gender-affirming care	Teach front-desk staff how to check-in a patient who uses a name that differs from their legal name and whose gender expression differs from the gender marker on their medical chart. This scenario is not uncommon for TGD people; in the US Transgender Survey, only 11% of TGD people had updated all records with the gender marker reflecting their gender identity.[3]
Determine how patients would like to be addressed	At registration, ask all patients what name they would like staff to use for them and what their pronouns are, and record this information in the electronic medical record, with patients' permission.
Establish and convey nondiscrimination policies that affirm TGD people	Post a nondiscrimination policy that includes gender identity and expression in the clinic. Information on how to report an instance of discrimination should also be included.
Adapt the physical environment to be inclusive of TGD people	Post signs that indicate patients and staff may use any restroom that matches their gender identity, and/or provide single-stall, all-gender restrooms. Invite staff members to include their pronouns in verbal and written introductions and to indicate them on identification badges.
Recognize and participate in community events of importance for TGD people	Acknowledge and celebrate the Transgender Day of Remembrance, the International Transgender Day of Visibility, Non-Binary Parents Day, Pride and other community events
Hire a diverse workforce that includes TGD people	Advertise open positions at TGD community organizations. Include language in job postings that TGD people are encouraged to apply.

a trauma-informed lens, clinicians can diminish expectations of discrimination and ultimately improve access for TGD people.

Understanding Clinical Care for Transgender and Gender Diverse People

A second step is to develop knowledge and expertise about clinical care for TGD people. Although TGD people largely require routine medical care that is delivered in an affirming manner, some aspects of care are unique. Foremost of these are the medical aspects of gender affirmation. Medical gender affirmation may include hormonal and/or surgical therapies.

Hormone Therapy

Hormone therapy is frequently sought for gender affirmation; of respondents to the 2015 US Transgender Survey, 78% desired hormonal therapy. The selection of hormonal therapies is typically tailored to an individual's goals, but common regimens for people assigned male sex at birth include oral, transdermal, or parenteral estradiol and an antiandrogen (eg, oral spironolactone or parenteral leuprolide); the latter is often omitted if the testes have been removed.[4] For people assigned female sex at birth, a common regimen is transdermal or parenteral testosterone.[4] Hormone therapy has well-established benefits for well-being for TGD people and is a cornerstone of gender affirmation for many.[5] Primary care clinicians should familiarize themselves with potential effects on general health of these treatments and recommended counseling, screening, and laboratory monitoring parameters.[5] These treatments also have predictable effects on sexual and reproductive function and anatomy, as summarized in **Table 2**. International guidelines recommend that clinicians providing these therapies counsel patients about the anticipated impacts on sexual function.[5]

Because exogenous testosterone may be teratogenic in pregnancy, people assigned female sex at birth who take testosterone and have vaginal or frontal sex with people whose bodies produce sperm should use contraception.[5]

These physiologic responses to hormone therapy should not be interpreted by clinicians to represent sexual dysfunction, because hormone therapy tends to improve sexual well-being, potentially by alleviating gender dysphoria.6 For example, in one study of 163 transgender men and women with a pre–post design, gender-affirming hormone therapy of at least 1 year's duration was associated with improvements in orgasm duration and satisfaction.[7]

Table 2
Anticipated effects on sexual and reproductive function and anatomy of common hormonal treatments

Patient Population	Effects
People assigned female sex at birth receiving testosterone	Amenorrhea[a] Atrophy of the vagina Clitoral enlargement
People assigned male sex at birth receiving estradiol and an antiandrogen (unless the testes have been removed)	Decreased libido Decreased penile erections Decreased testicular volume Reduction in sperm production

[a] Although testosterone may cause amenorrhea, it is not considered a reliable form of contraception.

From Hembree WC, Cohen-Kettenis PT, Gooren L, et al. Endocrine treatment of gender-dysphoric/gender-incongruent persons: an Endocrine Society clinical practice guideline. J Clin Endocrinol Metab. 2017;102(11):3869-3903.

Surgical Therapy

A range of surgical interventions are available for gender affirmation. Historically, only a fraction of TGD people were able to access surgery due to financial and insurance restrictions as well as gatekeeping by the medical system[3]; although insurance coverage has increased in some settings and the process of providing gender affirming therapies has shifted to an informed consent model in many institutions, many people have yet to receive the surgeries they seek. For people assigned male at birth, surgeries can include facial procedures, breast augmentation, orchiectomy, and vaginoplasty. For people assigned female at birth, surgeries may include facial procedures, mastectomy, hysterectomy, metoidioplasty (creation of a phallus from the clitoris, which has typically been enlarged by pre-treatment with testosterone), and/or phalloplasty; a list of potential surgical procedures is available in Appendix E of the World Professional Association of Transgender Health Standards of Care for the Health of Transgender and Gender Diverse People, Version 8.[5] Surgical techniques vary. For example, vaginoplasty may involve inversion of penile tissues or use of peritoneal or intestinal mucosa. Metoidioplasty may or may not include closure of the vaginal cavity.[5] It is thus important for clinicians to ask all patients about current anatomy (eg, whether the cervix, uterus, prostate, and vagina are present or absent) in order to recommend appropriate screening tests. Sometimes called an anatomic inventory, this approach is described in the sexual health screening chapter in this edition of the journal. For both groups, chest procedures are often termed "top" surgeries, and those on the genitals are called "bottom" surgeries. Because patients may vary in their desire for and receipt of surgeries, clinicians must avoid assumptions about anatomy when providing care and rather inquire in a non-judgmental fashion about the anatomy that is present as part of the anatomic inventory.[8]

Sexually Transmitted Infections Among Transgender and Gender Diverse People

Incidence and prevalence estimates for HIV and sexually transmitted infection (STIs) among TGD people most likely overestimate true values because they often rely on convenience samples; population-based studies which include TGD people are limited; and estimating an accurate denominator of TGD people is hampered by anti-transgender stigma (ie, people may not identify as TGD on surveys due to concerns about discrimination). However, some TGD populations may bear disproportionate burdens of STIs, including HIV. Transgender women, particularly transgender women of color, face a high prevalence of HIV. For example, in one study of transgender women in seven urban areas across the United States, the HIV prevalence was 42% overall and 62% among Black/African American transgender women.[9] Transgender women may also have high rates of bacterial STIs, including chlamydia and gonorrhea.[10,11] Transgender women are affected by multiple vulnerabilities that may increase their likelihood for STIs and HIV. These include higher-than-average rates of violence victimization, poverty, engagement in sex work, mental health conditions, and substance use disorders[3]; all of these factors stem ultimately from anti-transgender stigma and discrimination.

Data on STIs and HIV are more sparse among transgender men and nonbinary people. Some transgender men are sexually active with cisgender men and may engage in frontal (vaginal)-genital sex or receptive anal sex.[12] These transgender men who have sex with men (MSM) may face higher rates of STIs and HIV. A retrospective chart review from a large community health center in New York City evaluated rates of HIV screening and seroprevalence in 577 transgender men attending the center for routine hormone care. Forty-three percent had HIV screening while in care, with an HIV prevalence of 2.8%.[13] This prevalence was substantially higher than that previously documented in national data for transgender men. Transgender men reporting sex exclusively with cisgender men had a HIV prevalence of 11.1%, with an adjusted odds ratio of 10.58. Few if any data are available about STIs and HIV among nonbinary people; however, the self-reported HIV prevalence is 1% among nonbinary people assigned male sex at birth and 0.2% among nonbinary people assigned female sex at birth.[3] Although low, the prevalence of self-reported HIV among nonbinary people assigned male sex at birth exceeds that of the general population.

STIs can occur in surgically constructed genitalia, but data on the spectrum of clinical syndromes in these contexts are limited. Genital human papillomavirus, chlamydia, and gonorrhea have all been documented among people with a history of vaginoplasty.[14] Reports of STIs following phalloplasty are limited, though this is likely because the procedure is less common than vaginoplasty and because of limited data rather than because STIs cannot occur in that setting. We recommend clinicians consider STIs and test accordingly for any unexplained genital symptoms among TGD people who are sexually active at those anatomic sites. In addition, clinicians should recommend screening for STIs in accordance with national guidelines among sexually active TGD people, whether they have had gender-affirming genital surgeries or not.[15]

Providing Sexual Health Care for Transgender and Gender Diverse People

Applying key concepts about gender identity, strategies to make care gender affirming, and an understanding of hormonal and surgical therapies for TGD people, clinicians can take concrete steps to provide comprehensive sexual health care for TGD people (**Box 1**).

A first step is to obtain histories that are inclusive of all gender identities. As for all patients, eliciting a comprehensive sexual history is a key aspect of providing sexual health care. Please refer to the dedicated article on sexual history in this edition of the journal for more information. For an example of an inclusive, self-administered questionnaire to guide STI screening at a sexual health clinic, see ref.[16] For TGD patients, as for other patients, ensuring the history is free of assumptions about the gender identity and anatomy of sexual partners and the types of sexual activity is crucial. Because an individual's anatomy and how they use their body for sex cannot be presumed by knowing their gender identity or that of their partner(s), it is often helpful, as part of a comprehensive sexual history, to ask specifically about what types of sex a person has (eg, penile-frontal, penile-anal, and oral-anal). This information would guide sites of screening for chlamydia and gonorrhea and discussion about prevention

Box 1
Five steps for comprehensive sexual health care for transgender and gender diverse people

1. Elicit the sexual history in a manner that is inclusive of all gender identities
2. Mirror the language patients use to describe their identities and bodies
3. For STI testing that is anatomic site-specific (eg, gonorrhea and chlamydia screening), test based on current anatomy and sexual activity, and offer self-collection of specimens
4. Ensure that posters, pamphlets, Web sites, and other materials about sexual health include a range of gender identities and expressions
5. Colocate gender-affirming medical care with sexual health services

interventions such as HIV pre-exposure prophylaxis (PrEP). Clinicians should also explain to patients why the sexual history is being elicited, because some TGD people have faced unnecessary and voyeuristic questioning in medical settings previously.[3] To introduce the sexual history, clinicians could begin by saying, "I would now like to ask you some questions about your sexual history so that I can provide the best preventive care. Is that OK?"

Clinicians should be mindful of the nuances of eliciting sexual histories for all patients if framing sexual history questions around the sex/gender of partners or sexual orientation, particularly in populations where social-sexual networks are small. Phylogenetic analysis of newly diagnosed HIV infections among transgender women in Los Angeles county revealed that HIV transmission frequently occurred in multiple members of a social network linking cisgender men identifying as heterosexual and multiple transgender women.[17] Heterosexually identified cisgender men who have sex with transgender women may be considered "low risk" and not screened for HIV if clinicians ask only about sexual orientation; however, the addition of a follow-up questions asking about gender identities, anatomy, and sex practices would impact assessment of the likelihood of HIV and subsequent screening recommendations.

A second key step in sexual health care for TGD people is to mirror the language patients use to describe their identities and their bodies. For example, some transgender men may refer to the vagina as the front hole and call vaginal sex frontal sex.[12] Clinicians can ask about preferred terms with a question such as, "I generally use medical terms to describe body parts, such as penis and vagina. Are there different terms you use for your body that you would like me to use as well?"

Third, when screening for gonorrhea, chlamydia, and trichomoniasis, clinicians should adopt an approach based on current anatomy and sexual activity, as they would for cisgender people.[15] For example, a transgender man who engages in frontal sex with a cisgender man, a transgender woman who has had vaginoplasty and engages in vaginal sex with a cisgender man, and a cisgender woman who engages in vaginal sex with a cisgender man could all be screened for gonorrhea and chlamydia with a vaginal swab for nucleic acid amplification testing (NAAT). Although data to inform the performance of different specimen types in the setting of different genital surgeries are limited, NAATs for gonorrhea and chlamydia from all anatomic sites can be self-collected,[15] and self-testing for STIs is acceptable to and preferred by TGD people in a range of settings.[18–20] For example, in a study of self- versus clinician-collected of human papillomavirus screening among transgender men, most participants preferred self-collection.[19] For more information about gonorrhea, chlamydia, and trichomoniasis screening, please refer to the STI screening article in this edition of the journal.

In research, public health discourse, and sexual health care, transgender women have often historically been grouped with cisgender MSM, limiting awareness of their unique needs and diminishing their gender identities.[21] A fourth key step for improving sexual health care for TGD people is to avoid conflating transgender women and MSM. PrEP messaging, for example, has often focused on MSM. However, MSM-focused messages and materials may not reach transgender women and/or may be off-putting to them.[21] Ensuring that posters, brochures, and other materials about PrEP and other sexual health topics represent and are relevant to a diverse range of gender identities is crucial to help engage in care all who may benefit.

Finally, clinicians should aim to provide a range of services for TGD people beyond sexual health care. TGD people often desire obtaining PrEP or HIV treatment from the prescriber of their hormones, and colocating HIV prevention and care with gender-affirming care may improve HIV-related outcomes such as PrEP uptake.[22,23] Bundling sexual health care allows patients and clinicians to build on the success of and engagement in gender-affirming care. For example, patients initiating hormones often have frequent follow-up visits for clinical and laboratory monitoring; STI screening and/or PrEP could be offered at these visits. Engagement in sexual health care should never be a prerequisite for prescribing hormones, however. Even when gender-affirming and other care are not colocated, provision of gender-affirming care may positively impact other domains of health. For example, in an analysis of transgender people with HIV enrolled in Medicaid in New York, receipt of gender-affirming surgery was associated with substantial improvements in rates of viral suppression which were maintained years after an individual's last surgical procedure.[24]

SUMMARY

The World Health Organization defines sexual health as "physical, emotional, mental, and social well-being in relation to sexuality."[25] To help foster sexual health for TGD people in alignment with this expansive definition, sexual health care must be thoroughly and explicitly affirming of all gender identities and expressions. Clinicians can advance sexual health care for TGD people through strategies such as developing expertise in gender-affirming care, including its impacts on sexual health; communicating with patients in ways that do not convey assumptions about gender identity or anatomy; and colocating both sexual health and gender-affirming services. TGD people may face threats to sexual health, including stigma and discrimination as well as disproportionate burdens of STIs and HIV, but by embedding sexual health care within a gender-affirming environment, clinicians can counter these threats and help patients achieve the highest possible level of health.

CLINICS CARE POINTS

- TGD) people are those whose gender identities do not align with societal expectations based on their sex assigned at birth.
- Strategies to make care environments more welcoming for TGD people include training all staff members about key TGD concepts, asking all patients about their names and pronouns, establishing and displaying nondiscrimination policies that include gender identity and expression, providing access to single-stall or all-gender restrooms, and hiring a diverse clinical workforce that includes TGD people.
- Gender affirmation is a process through which TGD people make changes to live in alignment with their gender identities. Gender affirmation is unique to each individual but may include hormonal therapies (eg, estradiol with an antiandrogen or testosterone) and/or surgeries.
- Hormonal therapy may affect sexual function; in general, hormonal and surgical therapies tend to improve sexual function and satisfaction among TGD people.
- Some TGD populations, such as some sexually active transgender women, face an increased likelihood of STIs and HIV. Sexually transmitted infections (STIs) can affect surgically modified or constructed genitalia, and clinicians should consider STIs in the evaluation of unexplained genital symptoms in TGD people who are sexually active.
- To optimize sexual health care for TGD people, clinicians should elicit sexual histories that are inclusive of all gender identities, adopt an anatomy-based approach to STI screening, offer self-swabbing for gonorrhea and chlamydia nucleic acid amplification tests, and colocate sexual health and gender-affirming services.

DISCLOSURE

K. L. Ard has received in-kind research support from Binx Health. A.C Demidont and A MacDonald-Ly are full-time employees (HIV Medical Affairs) with Gilead Sciences, Inc.

REFERENCES

1. Meerwijk E, Sevelius JM. Transgender population size in the United States: a meta-regression of population-based probability samples. Am J Pub Health 2017;107:e1–8.
2. LGBTQIA+ glossary of terms for health care teams. National LGBTQIA+ Health Education Center. The Fenway Institute; 2020. Available at: https://www.lgbtqiahealtheducation.org/publication/lgbtqia-glossary-of-terms-for-health-care-teams/. Accessed 12 July 2023.
3. James SE, Herman JL, Rankin S, et al. The report of the 2015 U.S. Transgender Survey. Washington, DC: National Center for Transgender Equality; 2016. Available at: https://transequality.org/sites/default/files/docs/usts/USTS-Full-Report-Dec17.pdf. Accessed 6 July 2023.
4. Hembree WC, Cohen-Kettenis PT, Gooren L, et al. Endocrine treatment of gender-dysphoric/gender-incongruent persons: an Endocrine Society clinical practice guideline. J Clin Endocrinol Metab 2017;102(11):3869–903.
5. Coleman E, Radix A, Bouman WP, et al. Standards of care for the health of transgender and gender diverse people, version 8. Int J Trans Health 2022;23(S1):S1–260.
6. Murad MH, Elamin MB, Bacia MZ, et al. Hormonal therapy and sex reassignment: a systematic review and meta-analysis of quality of life and psychosocial outcomes. Clin Endocrinol 2010;72(2):214–31.
7. Zaliznyak M, Lauzon M, Stelmar J, et al. Effects of gender-affirming hormone therapy on orgasm function of transgender men and women: a long-term follow up. Urology 2023;174:86–91.
8. Grasso C, Goldhammer H, Thompson J, et al. Optimizing gender-affirming medical care through anatomical inventories, clinical decision support, and population health management in electronic health record systems. J Am Med Inform Assoc 2021;28(11):2531–5.
9. HIV and transgender people: HIV prevalence. Centers for Disease Control and Prevention. HIV Surveillance Special Report 2021. Accessed 12 Jul 2023. Available at: https://www.cdc.gov/hiv/group/gender/transgender/hiv-prevalence.html.
10. Pitasi MA, Kerani RP, Kohn R, et al. Chlamydia, gonorrhea, and human immunodeficiency virus infection among transgender women and transgender men attending clinics that provide sexually transmitted disease services in six US cities: results from the Sexually Transmitted Disease Surveillance Network. Sex Transm Dis 2019;46(2):112–7.
11. Van Gerwen OT, Jani A, Long DM, et al. Prevalence of sexually transmitted infections and human immunodeficiency virus in transgender persons: a systematic review. Transgend Health 2020;5(2):90–103.
12. Reisner SL, Pletta DR, Pardee DJ, et al. Digital-assisted self-interview of HIV or sexually transmitted infection risk behaviors in transmasculine adults: development and field testing of the transmasculine sexual health assessment. JMIR Public Health Surveill 2023;9:e40503.
13. Radix AE, Larson EL, Harris AB, Chiasson MA. HIV prevalence among transmasculine individuals at a New York City Community Health Centre: a cross-sectional study. J Int AIDS Soc 2022;25(Suppl 5):e25981.

14. Van Gerwen OT, Aryanpour Z, Selph JP, et al. Anatomical and sexual health considerations among transfeminine individuals who have undergone vaginoplasty: a review. Int J STD AIDS 2022;33(2):106–13.
15. Workowski KA, Bachmann LH, Chan PA, et al. Sexually transmitted infections treatment guidelines, 2021. MMWR Recomm Rep (Morb Mortal Wkly Rep) 2021;70(4):1–192.
16. Tordoff DM, Dombrowski JC, Ramchandani MC, et al. Trans-inclusive sexual health questionnaire to improve human immunodeficiency virus/sexually transmitted infection (STI) care for transgender patients: anatomic site-specific STI prevalence and screening. Clin Infect Dis 2023;76(3):e736–43.
17. Ragonnet-Cronin M, Hu YW, Morris SR, et al. HIV transmission networks among transgender women in Los Angeles County, CA, USA: a phylogenetic analysis of surveillance data. Lancet HIV 2019;6(3):e164–72.
18. McCartney DJ, Pinheiro TF, Gomez JL, et al. Acceptability of self-sampling for etiological diagnosis of mucosal sexually transmitted infections (STIs) among transgender women in a longitudinal cohort study in Sao Paolo, Brazil. Braz J Infect Dis 2022;26(3):102356.
19. Reisner SL, Deutsch MB, Peitzmeier SM, et al. Test performance and acceptability of self- versus provider-collected swabs for high-risk HPV DNA testing in female-to-male transmasculine patients. PLoS One 2018;13(3):e0190172.
20. Hiransuthikul A, Janamnuaysook R, Himma L, et al. Acceptability and satisfaction towards self-collection for chlamydia and gonorrhoea testing among transgender women in Tangerine Clinic, Thailand: shifting towards the new normal. J Int AIDS Soc 2021;24(9):e25801.
21. Sevelius JM, Keatley J, Calma N, et al. 'I am not a man': Trans-specific barriers and facilitators to PrEP acceptability among transgender women. Glob Public Health 2016;11(7–8):1060–75.
22. Sevelius JM, Deutsch MB, Grant R. The future of PrEP among transgender women: the critical role of gender affirmation in research and clinical practices. J Int AIDS Soc 2016;19(7Suppl6):21105.
23. Sevelius JM, Glidden DV, Deutsch M, et al. Uptake, retention, and adherence to pre-exposure prophylaxis (PrEP) in TRIUMPH: A peer-led PrEP demonstration project for transgender communities in Oakland and Sacramento, California. J Acquir Immune Defic Syndr 2021;88(S1):S27–38.
24. Rodriguez-Hart C, Zhao G, Goldstein Z, et al. Gender affirming surgery associated with high viral suppression among transgender PWH. Conference on Retroviruses and Opportunistic Infections 2021. Abstract 107.
25. Sexual health. World Health Organization. 2023. Accessed 13 Jul 2023. Available at: https://www.who.int/health-topics/sexual-health#tab=tab_2.

On The Horizon

Novel Approaches to Sexually Transmitted Infection Prevention

Chase A. Cannon, MD, MPH[a,*],
Stephanie E. McLaughlin, MD, MPH[b],
Meena S. Ramchandani, MD, MPH[a]

KEYWORDS

• STI prevention • Doxycycline PEP • Meningococcal vaccine • Point of care testing

KEY POINTS

- Doxycycline post-exposure prophylaxis is an emerging strategy which appears effective for reducing bacterial sexually transmitted infections (STIs) in men who have sex with men and transgender women with a history of STI.
- Evolving evidence suggests immunization with meningococcal outer membrane vesicle vaccines may confer cross-protection against gonorrhea.
- Self-sampling and point of care testing for STI are increasingly being utilized across clinical and non-clinical sites and may increase uptake and acceptability of STI screening.

INTRODUCTION

In the face of burgeoning gonorrhea (GC), chlamydia (CT), and infectious syphilis epidemics, national efforts to decrease incidence of sexually transmitted infections (STIs) have focused on increasing awareness, testing populations based on individual risk or local epidemiology, and early treatment of incident infections. Despite these efforts, strategies for population-level STI control have been few and limited in their effectiveness. The Centers for Disease Control and Prevention (CDC) and the United States Department of Health and Human Services released a federal implementation plan for STI prevention from 2021 to 2025 focused on facilitating accelerated progress in STI innovation and research.[1] Key strategies include using antibiotic post-exposure prophylaxis, exploring existing and novel vaccines for prevention, and leveraging point of care and self-testing for earlier detection and diagnosis of STI. Geared toward

[a] Department of Medicine, Division of Allergy and Infectious Diseases, University of Washington, Public Health – Seattle & King County, 325 9th Avenue, Box 359777, Seattle, WA 98104, USA; [b] University of Washington, 325 9th Avenue, Box 359777, Seattle, WA 98104, USA
* Corresponding author.
E-mail address: ccannon5@uw.edu

Med Clin N Am 108 (2024) 403–418
https://doi.org/10.1016/j.mcna.2023.10.003

general practitioners, this review highlights some of the latest research on selected innovative approaches to STI prevention either currently available or under development for future use that may impact clinical practice for providers who care for adolescents or adults at risk for STI.

ANTIMICROBIAL PROPHYLAXIS FOR STI

Biomedical prophylaxis for STI prevention is a strategy that has gained popularity in the past 10 to 15 years since the initial approval of emtricitabine-tenofovir disoproxil fumarate as human immunodeficiency virus (HIV) pre-exposure prophylaxis (PrEP) by the US Food and Drug Administration (FDA) in 2012. Several studies conducted in recent years (**Table 1**) have now shown that use of event-driven doxycycline post-exposure prophylaxis (doxy-PEP) in men who have sex with men (MSM) and transgender women (TGW) is efficacious in reducing bacterial STI incidence.[2–4]

The first major trial to evaluate doxy-PEP occurred within a parent study of event-driven HIV PrEP among HIV-negative MSM in France. Men in the trial were randomized 1:1 to receive either open-label doxycycline PEP or no prophylaxis.[2] Those taking doxy-PEP saw a 47% relative risk reduction (RRR) in time to first incident STI—primarily due to decreases in syphilis and CT.[2] Gastrointestinal side effects were more common in the doxy-PEP arm, but few participants (7%) discontinued doxycycline due to adverse events.

Based on these data, investigators in the United States initiated a larger randomized controlled trial (RCT) including MSM and TGW who were living with HIV or HIV-negative and taking HIV PrEP in Seattle and San Francisco. Participants were also randomized to standard of care or to receive open-label doxycycline.[3] In contrast to the French study, the US DoxyPEP trial showed a 65% RRR in all 3 bacterial STI (GC, CT, and syphilis) at 12 months.[3] Though doxy-PEP participants overall took more doxycycline compared to the standard care arm, they also used 50% less ceftriaxone—a much broader spectrum antibiotic. Rare adverse events including 1 instance of transaminitis, and side effects of diarrhea and headache were reported; only 2% of study participants discontinued the drug.

Shortly after enrollment in the US trial began, the French research group from the original open-label doxy PEP substudy initiated the DOXYVAC trial employing a factorial design to randomize MSM on PrEP with a history of bacterial STI to receive doxycycline versus no doxycycline in combination with 4CMenB vaccine versus no vaccine. Final results from the study are not yet published, but preliminary data were presented at an international scientific conference in spring of 2023. Investigators found that despite high baseline gonococcal resistance to tetracyclines in France, this second trial also showed independent benefit of doxy-PEP for CT and syphilis (combined 84% risk reduction) as well as GC (51% risk reduction).[4]

Finally, a study conducted in Kenya randomized cisgender women taking HIV PrEP to receive open-label doxycycline versus standard of care (quarterly STI testing and treatment). Of note, the study's primary aim was not to evaluate all 3 bacterial STI given that (1) syphilis is uncommon among women in sub-Saharan Africa and (2) doxy-PEP was not expected to impact GC incidence since tetracycline resistance in *Neisseria gonorrhoeae* (NG) is nearly ubiquitous in Kenya. The trial's manuscript is not yet published, but preliminary results for both doxy-PEP efficacy and adherence were presented at 2 international scientific conferences in 2023. Investigators found no significant difference in CT incidence between the doxy-PEP and control arms.[5] While there were no new cases of HIV diagnosed in the trial—suggesting at least moderate adherence to PrEP—subsequent hair analyses of participants in the doxycycline

Table 1
Clinical trial evidence for doxycycline post-exposure prophylaxis (doxy-PEP)

Clinical Trial	Study Participants		Doxycycline Dosing Strategy	Relative Risk Reduction (95% CI) for Doxy-PEP	Absolute Risk Reduction for Doxy-PEP	Summary of Evidence for Clinical Practice
IPERGAY (France, 2015–2016)	232 MSM on PrEP		200 mg once PO within 24–72 h after condomless sex; maximum of 3 doses per week	47%[a] (15%–67%)	32 per 100 person-years[a]	Proof of concept for doxy-PEP's efficacy for reducing CT and syphilis in MSM.
DoxyPEP (US, 2020–2022)	501 MSM & TGW with recent bacterial STI	PWH (n = 174)	200 mg once PO within 24–72 h after condomless sex; maximum of 1 dose per day	52% (17%–72%)	18.7% per quarter	Doxy-PEP is efficacious for preventing syphilis, GC and CT for MSM and TGW with history of prior STI.
		PrEP (n = 327)		66% (49%–77%)	21.2% per quarter	
DOXYVAC (France, 2021–2022)	502 MSM on PrEP with recent bacterial STI		200 mg once PO within 24–72 h after condomless sex; maximum of 3 doses per week	84%[a] (70%–92%)	30 per 100 person-years[a]	Further evidence supporting doxy-PEP's efficacy for preventing syphilis, GC and CT in MSM.
dPEP (Kenya, 2020–2022)	449 cisgender women on PrEP		200 mg once PO within 24–72 h after condomless sex; maximum of 1 dose per day	12% ($P = .51$)	9 total GC/CT infections at 12 mo	Based on available evidence at this time, doxy-PEP is not recommended for preventing STI in cisgender women.

Abbreviations: CI, confidence interval; CT, chlamydia; GC, gonorrhea; HIV, pre-exposure prophylaxis; MSM, men who have sex with men; orally, PrEP; PO, per os; PWH, people with HIV; STI, sexually transmitted infections; TGW, transgender women.

[a] Risk reduction estimate is for chlamydia and syphilis only.

Data compiled from Molina, Lancet 2018; Luetkemeyer and colleagues, NEJM 2023; Molina, CROI 2023; Stewart, CROI 2023.

arm suggested that low adherence to doxy-PEP may have explained the null effect seen for STI prevention.[6] Additional qualitative analyses are ongoing to understand what contributed to suboptimal adherence in the study and explore how doxy-PEP may impact STI prevention approaches for cisgender women. Studies to evaluate doxycycline pre-exposure prophylaxis (doxy-PrEP) as a bacterial STI prevention strategy in MSM and TGW are also underway in Australia and Canada[7–9]; results are not yet available.

Although the clinical trials described earlier have provided evidence supporting use of doxy-PEP in certain populations, there are important considerations to weigh as doxy-PEP is implemented into clinical practice (**Table 2**). Doxycycline is a second-generation tetracycline first approved by the FDA in 1967[10] that is generally safe, well-tolerated, has a long half-life of 20 hours, and high bioavailability. Use during pregnancy is generally not recommended due to undetermined risk about staining of primary teeth.[11] Doxycycline has a broad antimicrobial spectrum and activity against several bacteria and parasites including a number of bacterial STI pathogens. Side effects from doxycycline may include gastrointestinal upset (nausea, vomiting, and diarrhea), risk for pill esophagitis, and photosensitivity.

Current uncertainties about doxy-PEP include whether by reducing the rates of GC, CT, and syphilis in MSM or TGW the intervention will lead to lower numbers of complicated syphilis (eg, neurosyphilis) or otherwise have a broader impact on population-level STI rates (see **Table 2**). As doxycycline can be used to treat syphilis or CT or as part of treatment for *Mycoplasma genitalium*, it is unknown to what extent doxy-PEP may function as subtherapeutic treatment for these infections. If this is the case, there are questions about whether having a lower bacterial burden could impact the minimum threshold of detection for current nucleic acid amplification tests or whether treatment could impact immune responses and hence serologic diagnostics for syphilis, thereby making the diagnosis of incident STI more challenging on doxy-PEP. Answering these questions will likely require either targeted prospective studies or enhanced STI surveillance systems.

With continued use, there are possible risks of inducing antimicrobial resistance (AMR) and possible effects on the microbiome of both individuals and populations. For example, as doxycycline has activity against *Staphylococcus aureus* and *Streptococcus pneumoniae*, there are concerns that use of doxy-PEP at the population level could lead to higher prevalence of tetracycline resistance in these organisms. The US DoxyPEP trial found that while *S. aureus* colonization decreased in the doxy-PEP arm, isolation of doxycycline-resistant *S aureus* increased 8% at 12 months.[3] Studies have found both positive and negative associations between chronic diseases (eg, type 1 diabetes or asthma) and bacteria in the gut microbiota that are affected by doxycycline,[12] raising concern about whether doxy-PEP could impact their incidence in the future. As a surrogate evaluation of doxycycline's effect on the microbiome, the DOXYVAC trial measured presence of extended-spectrum beta-lactamses *E. coli* from anal swabs and found baseline rates were around 30% and increased to 35% to 40% in both groups by month 12.[4] AMR in NG is concerning as most classes of antibiotics used to treat GC are no longer effective due to resistance. One mathematical model suggests that if doxy-PEP use increases in the population, the incidence and prevalence of GC will decrease while resistant strains could predominate, subsequently minimizing the overall effect of doxy-PEP for GC prevention within 10 years.[13] Tetracycline resistance has never been described for CT or syphilis, and it is unknown whether this could occur in the future. Leveraging existing surveillance systems and proactively monitoring for resistance in various STI organisms must be a component of doxy-PEP implementation.

Table 2
Key considerations for counseling about doxycycline post-exposure prophylaxis (doxy-PEP)

Benefits or "Pros" for Doxy-PEP	Potential Adverse Effects or "Cons" Against Doxy-PEP	Unknowns About Doxy-PEP Use
• Substantially reduces bacterial STI risk (NNT = 5) in certain MSM and TGW • Doxycycline is cheap, safe, and generally well tolerated • May reduce STI-related stigma • PEP involves less use of antibiotics than PrEP • Reduced ceftriaxone use by 50% in DoxyPEP trial[3]	• Side effects: photosensitivity, GI upset, risk for pill esophagitis • May eventually induce resistance in *Neisseria gonorrhoeae* • May increase resistance in *Staph. aureus*, *Strep. pneumoniae*, and other bystander organisms • Could impact ability to diagnose new STI (syphilis, *Mycoplasma genitalium*, etc.)	• Unclear whether doxy-PEP will reduce STI at population level • Unknown whether doxy-PEP will reduce morbidity associated with cases of complicated syphilis (eg, neurosyphilis) • Short and long-term effect on microbiome in the individual and population? • Through possible microbiome changes, could doxy-PEP increase risk for diabetes and other chronic illnesses?

Abbreviations: MSM, men who have sex with men; NNT, number needed to treat; PrEP, pre-exposure prophylaxis; STI, sexually transmitted infections; TGW, transgender women.

For primary care providers wanting to use doxy-PEP in their clinical practice, it is important to first recognize which populations were studied and for whom it may be beneficial. Although this still represents off-label use, current evidence supports the use of doxy-PEP in select MSM and TGW, especially those diagnosed with a bacterial STI in the prior year (see **Table 1**), and the intervention is available for any provider to prescribe now. Doxy-PEP is not currently recommended for cisgender women due to lack of efficacy in the primary clinical trial. Data are insufficient to support prescribing for other populations including MSM without a history of STI in the prior year, cisgender men who have sex with women and other gender diverse populations. Offering doxy-PEP to populations beyond those studied in primary trials may be considered on a case-by-case basis.

Providers wanting to offer doxy-PEP should review which patients may meet criteria and plan to broach the topic with eligible persons by providing a fact sheet or initiating direct conversation at a clinic visit. When discussing doxy-PEP, current evidence, benefits, risks, and unknowns should be reviewed and the choice to prescribe should result from shared decision-making. Jurisdictions in California, King County, Washington, and other clinics and organizations[14,15] have developed their own recommendations, clinical guidelines, and patient fact sheets, which may be reviewed and adapted for a provider's clinical practice. These local guidelines include details on the dosage, instructions, number of refills, preferred ICD-10 diagnosis code, and approaches to counseling. Final guidance on doxy-PEP from the CDC is expected in the near future; interested providers should check the CDC's website for details.

SELF-SAMPLING FOR SEXUALLY TRANSMITTED INFECTION

When nucleic acid amplification tests (NAAT) were first validated as a primary diagnostic method for GC and CT, specimens were to be collected by clinicians only. The process of clinicians collecting samples from "sensitive" areas, particularly for vaginal and rectal specimens, may be intrusive and uncomfortable. Many patients prefer the comfort and privacy associated with collecting their own samples.[16,17] Self-collection of specimens—a process by which a patient is instructed on how to collect their own swabs—is now available and often the standard, preferred approach for STI testing, at least for asymptomatic individuals.[18–20]

Ample evidence shows that self-collection of specimens is valid from a scientific and programmatic standpoint and easy to implement in clinical and nonclinical settings. The sensitivity and specificity of self-collected versus clinician-collected vaginal and urine GC, CT, and trichomonas NAAT specimens have been thoroughly evaluated across populations and proven to be equivalent.[21,22] A World Health Organization (WHO)-sponsored meta-analysis of STI services showed that programs offering self-collection of samples experienced a nearly 200% higher uptake of STI screening across populations.[23]

For several GC/CT NAAT, the FDA allows for self-sampling (eg, self-collected vaginal or urine specimens) in a healthcare setting where medical instruction, supervision, and assistance are readily available.[24] These can be ordered directly by the provider to be collected in their clinic or via a third-party laboratory for self-collection in their facility. In contrast to pharyngeal and rectal GC/CT specimens that are FDA approved for clinician collection, self-collection of extragenital specimens for GC/CT NAAT currently requires that the testing laboratory conduct an internal validation to ensure results are adequate between sample types.[21] This process should occur according to requirements of the laboratory's regulatory agency, and once complete, is sufficient for providers to begin implementing self-collection of samples in their clinics. Many health systems including HIV and municipal sexual health clinics have completed such validations for self-collected extragenital GC/CT specimens and made this method standard practice.[25]

Several commercial laboratories, academic centers, and clinics have validated home-based STI testing programs allowing patients to collect GC and CT samples at home and mail them to an approved laboratory.[26,27] Validation of self-collected samples for syphilis testing is also possible; however, laboratory-developed testing for syphilis is more complex given that liquid blood must be collected and stored for shipping in either microtainer tubes or onto dried blood spot cards. Since 2 serologic syphilis tests (often including a rapid plasma regain) are required to make a diagnosis, limited blood volume remains a challenge for broader implementation.

Point of Care Testing for sexually transmitted infection

Point of care tests (POCT) are helpful to diagnose CT, GC, and trichomoniasis at the site of clinical care or treatment initiation, improve clinical decision-making, and prevent onward transmission or complications from untreated STI. While the Gram stain, darkfield microscopy and microscopy of vaginal secretions ("wet mount") are historical mainstays for STI diagnosis, this section will review newer generation POCT for STI diagnosis including NAAT, antigen, and antibody tests. No point of care self-testing platforms are currently available for patients to perform and interpret results on their own. However, **Table 3** details several POCT platforms currently available that can be ordered and used in clinical settings by providers for NG, CT, or TV; in the future others may become available. Select test characteristics are further outlined in **Table 4**.[21,28–30]

A POCT which detects CT and NG has been incorporated into several healthcare settings. Studies have shown implementation of this POCT reduced inappropriate overtreatment for patients without infections[31–34] and increased the proportion of adolescents receiving same-day CT and NG treatment in Los Angeles and New Orleans.[35] Rapid and inexpensive antigen-based POCT for *C. trachomatis* are available; however, the sensitivity of these tests is lower than NAAT options.[29] Multiple platforms for detecting trichomoniasis are also available that produce quick results (**Table 3**).

Early detection, diagnosis, and rapid treatment of syphilis are important, especially among surging rates of syphilis nationally.[36,38] Two primary POCT for syphilis are FDA cleared, Clinical Laboratory Improvement Amendments (CLIA) waived, and available to use in the United States: 1 for syphilis alone and 1 dual HIV/syphilis assay. The sensitivity and specificity of these tests are detailed in **Table 4**. Both options use fingerstick whole-blood specimens and return results in less than 20 minutes. Since these tests detect treponemal-specific antibodies, they are useful as a screening tool in persons without a history of syphilis, and in the case of the dual HIV/syphilis test, also for those who may be at risk for HIV acquisition. Laboratory-based testing including non-treponemal (or lipoidal) antibodies is required to confirm any diagnosis of syphilis or HIV regardless of the POCT used. Few nontreponemal POCT has been evaluated in pilot studies,[38] but none are commercially available at present.

Important limitations of POCT include the need for personnel training (particularly for non-CLIA-waived platforms), restricted approval for few sample types, and prohibitive cost of the systems and tests. Several POCT for STI are under development that aim to improve diagnostic accuracy, reduce cost, and detect markers of antimicrobial resistance. In the United States, there are no commercially available POCT to detect *M genitalium* or drug resistance for STI pathogens, but such assays are in developmental phases.[39,40]

Table 3
Examples of currently available point of care tests for diagnosing NG, CT or TV

Test and Manufacturer	Type of Assay	Pathogens Detected	Time to Results	Approved Anatomic Sites	Comments
GeneXpert CT/NG (Cepheid)	PCR	CT, NG	Within 90 min	FDA cleared; not CLIA waived for urine, endocervical, vaginal, rectal, and pharyngeal specimens. Self-collected swabs allowed for some anatomic sites.	Shown to be acceptable and feasible in various healthcare settings and locations[63,64]
binx *io* CT/NG (binx health)	PCR	CT, NG	Within 30 min	FDA cleared and CLIA waived for female vaginal and male urine specimens[30,65–67]	Table-top system is approx. size of a conventional toaster
Visby Sexual Health Test (Visby Medical)	PCR	CT, NG, TV	Within 30 min	FDA cleared and CLIA waived for clinician- or self-obtained vaginal samples[68,69]	Small, compact device that fits in the hand
Xpert TV (Cepheid)	PCR	TV	Within 90 min	FDA cleared; not CLIA waived for female and male urine specimens, endocervical swabs, patient-collected vaginal swabs[29,70]	Useful for symptomatic and asymptomatic infections
Solana Trichomonas (Quidel)	PCR	TV	Within 35 min	FDA cleared; not CLIA waived for clinician-collected vaginal swabs and female urine specimens[71]	Useful for symptomatic and asymptomatic infections
OSOM Trichomonas Rapid Test (Sekisui Diagnostics)	Rapid antigen	TV	Within 10 min	FDA cleared and CLIA waived for vaginal swabs or vaginal wet mounts[71]	Sensitivity ranging from 83%-96% and specificity 95%.[72]

Abbreviations: CLIA, clinical laboratory improvement amendments; CT, chlamydia trachomatis; NG, neisseria gonorrhoeae; PCR, polymerase chain reaction; STI, sexually transmitted infections; TV, trichomonas vaginalis.
Note: Regulatory approval information as of August 2023.

Table 4
Sensitivity and specificity of currently available, FDA-cleared point of care tests (POCT) for STI

NG/CT/TV Nucleic Acid Amplification Tests	Sensitivity (%)	Specificity (%)
Cepheid: GeneXpert CT/NG[a]	86–99	99–100
binx health: binx io CT/NG[a]	93%–100%	99–100
Visby Medical: Visby Sexual Health test[a]	97–99	97–99
Cepheid: Xpert TV[a]	96–100	99
Quidel: Solana Trichomonas[a]	92–100	98–99
Syphilis diagnostic tests[37]		
Syphilis Health Check	50–100	88–100
Chembio Dual Path Platform HIV/Syphilis Assay	47–97	100

Abbreviations: CT, chlamydia trachomatis; NG, neisseria gonorrhoeae; STI, sexually transmitted infections; TV, trichomonas vaginalis.

[a] Sensitivity and specificities differ by detected pathogen and/or anatomic site.

VACCINES FOR SEXUALLY TRANSMITTED INFECTION

Early Promise of a Gonorrhea Vaccine

Modeling studies project that even a modestly effective gonococcal vaccine could have substantial impact on disease burden and help to achieve the goal of primary prevention for GC.[41] Development of a gonococcus-specific vaccine, however, has proven difficult since NG can change its outer membrane antigens to evade the immune system, which makes selection of a single antigen target for candidate vaccines challenging. Given that *Neisseria meningitidis*, a related bacterium in the same genus and the causative agent of epidemic meningococcal meningitis, shares similar antigens with NG, researchers began to explore using certain meningococcal vaccines to induce gonococcal cross-protection. Indeed, subsequent research validated the hypothesis that existing 4CMenB outer membrane vesicle (OMV) vaccines can provide protection again GC.[42–44]

Several epidemiologic studies have confirmed a decrease in GC after deployment of existing meningococcal vaccines. A retrospective review of epidemiologic data in Norway reported a decrease in GC cases among adolescents between 1988 and 1992 after the meningitis B OMV vaccine (MenBvac) was deployed.[45] In New Zealand, a case-control study demonstrated a vaccine efficacy of 31% against incident GC in individuals who received the MeNZB OMV vaccine compared to controls, even after adjustment for sex, ethnicity, geographic area, and economic status.[42] Data from a matched cohort study at Kaiser Permanente in Southern California showed that adjusted GC rates were 46% lower in those receiving the 4CMenB OMV vaccine Bexsero compared to controls receiving the MenACWY vaccine (which is not expected to induce gonococcal cross-protection).[46] Finally, preliminary reports from the French DOXYVAC trial also described a reduction of GC in its 4CMenB vaccine arm.[4] However, investigators later presented additional unpublished data at an international scientific conference demonstrating that this initial effect for GC prevention did not reach statistical significance and concluded that the 4CMenB vaccine should not yet be used for primary GC prevention.[47]

Likely due to the mixed evidence to date, major health organizations, including the CDC and WHO, have yet to recommend broad use of meningococcal vaccines to prevent GC. Bexsero and VA-MENGOC-BC are licensed and available in certain countries, but high cost, limited supply, and the lack of sufficient data to support regulatory approval for primary GC prevention remain barriers to use. For adolescents and young adults through age 25 and at risk for STI, Bexsero is FDA approved to prevent invasive meningococcal disease and could provide the added potential benefit of GC prevention. Primary care providers might consider off-label use of Bexsero in the United States for older adults on a case-by-case basis.

Four RCT are ongoing to evaluate the effectiveness of meningococcal B OMV vaccines for GC prevention: a phase 2 multi-site US trial (NCT04350138), *MenGO* (Australia),[48] *GoGoVax* (Australia, NCT04415424), and "*B Part of it NT*" (Australia, NCT04398849). In June 2023, the FDA approved "fast track" status of a novel investigational gonococcal vaccine based on positive results and safety data from the multi-country phase 1 portion of an industry-sponsored, first-time-in-human study.[49] Results from these trials may eventually add to evidence supporting approval of 1 or more vaccines for GC prevention.

Progress Toward Syphilis and Chlamydia Vaccines

Despite early progress with vaccine-induced protection in the rabbit model,[50] the ability to generate durable sterilizing immunity to *Treponema pallidum* has remained elusive and correlates of immune protection remain ill-defined in rabbits and humans.[51] Nonetheless, recently described animal-independent culture techniques[52,53] and advances in genomic methods[54] for antigen discovery provide hope to syphilis vaccine researchers. Studies combining outer membrane protein antigens with novel T-cell stimulating adjuvants are ongoing in rabbits to better define human vaccine antigen candidates.[55] Though the field is evolving rapidly, we likely remain years away from an effective syphilis vaccine for use in primary care. In contrast, a CT vaccine may be closer at hand; 1 prospective vaccine has successfully cleared phase 1 human trials[56], and efforts to move it along the development pipeline are underway.

The Future of Human Papillomavirus Vaccination

Though the development of highly effective human papillomavirus (HPV) vaccines represents a great success in the field of STI prevention, uptake, and completion of the 3-injection series of Gardasil-9 for HPV prevention have been suboptimal. Multiple strategies have aimed to improve HPV vaccine uptake including reducing the number of doses needed to complete a series. Clinical trial data show that immunogenicity in adolescents is equivalent or higher after 2 doses of HPV vaccine when compared to traditional 3-dose regimens,[57] leading to the recommendation of a 2-dose HPV vaccine series for adolescents aged less than 15 years that may improve vaccine uptake and coverage.[57,58] Studies have shown that even a single dose of HPV vaccine is immunogenic, and that although antibody titers are lower than in persons who received multiple doses, HPV seropositivity persists at 24 months after a single-dose vaccination.[59–61] As a result, single-dose HPV vaccination is now endorsed by the WHO[60,61] and a similar recommendation could follow in the United States after completion of a double-blinded, non-inferiority RCT evaluating single and 2-dose regimens.[62] The HPV vaccine is now also approved for previously unvaccinated adults aged 27 to 45. Vaccination is recommended for all older adults who are immunocompromised and can be considered in others based on a cost-benefit discussion.[58] Innovative clinical trials to evaluate the immunogenicity of intradermal fractional doses (0.1 mL, or one-fifth of standard 0.5-mL HPV vaccine doses) of bivalent and nonavalent HPV vaccines are ongoing (NCT04235257). If successful, the strategy could impact future vaccination schedules for older adults and expand vaccine supply in areas with decreased access.

SUMMARY

Rates of STI, especially cases of infectious and congenital syphilis, are increasing in the United States. Several evidence-based strategies for STI prevention are available to implement now including doxy-PEP for MSM and transgender women with a history of prior STI, and employing self-collection of genital and extragenital samples and point of care platforms to improve the acceptability, uptake, and access of STI testing for key populations. Evidence supports the immunogenicity of shorter 1-dose or 2-dose HPV vaccine series and may improve coverage in adolescents and young adults. The potential utility of meningococcal vaccines against *N gonorrhoeae* is being explored, but mixed evidence to date has not yet supported widespread use. Research to develop a syphilis vaccine is ongoing and a candidate CT vaccine may move to late phase human trials within the next several years. Focusing on effective implementation of current evidence-based strategies will be the key to maximizing future STI prevention efforts.

CLINICS CARE POINTS

- Doxycycline post-exposure prophylaxis is an evidence-based strategy to prevent bacterial sexually transmitted infection (STI) in men who have sex with men and transgender women with a history of STI that should be presented to eligible patients along with potential risks and unknowns.
- Evidence supports that self-collection of genital and extragenital samples for gonorrhea and chlamydia testing is equivalent to clinician collection and can increase uptake of STI testing in key populations.
- Several point of care tests (POCT) for STI are available and produce rapid results for gonorrhea, chlamydia, syphilis and trichomonas. Implementation of POCT can improve clinical decision making and facilitate quicker and more targeted treatment of STI.
- Meningococcal B vaccine has shown some promise for gonorrhea prevention, but widespread use for this purpose is not yet recommended. Clinical trials to further evaluate effectiveness are ongoing.
- Clinical data support HPV vaccination as a single or 2-dose series, which may increase acceptability and uptake among adolescents and young adults.

DISCLOSURE

The authors have no commercial or financial conflicts of interest to declare.

REFERENCES

1. Sexually Transmitted Infections National Strategic Plan for the United States: 2021–2025 | National Prevention Information Network | Connecting public health professionals with trusted information and each other. https://npin.cdc.gov/publication/sexually-transmitted-infections-national-strategic-plan-united-states-2021%E2%80%932025.
2. Molina JM, Charreau I, Chidiac C, et al. Post-exposure prophylaxis with doxycycline to prevent sexually transmitted infections in men who have sex with men: an open-label randomised substudy of the ANRS IPERGAY trial. Lancet Infect Dis 2018;18(3):308–17.
3. Luetkemeyer AF, Donnell D, Dombrowski JC, et al. Postexposure doxycycline to prevent bacterial sexually transmitted infections. N Engl J Med 2023;388(14):1296–306.

4. Molina JM. Anrs 174 DOXYVAC: an open-label randomized trial to prevent STIs in MSM on PrEP. Seattle, Washington: CROI; 2023. Presented at.
5. Stewart J. Doxycycline postexposure prophylaxis for prevention of STIs among cisgender women. Seattle, Washington: CROI; 2023. Presented at.
6. Stewart J. Adherence to doxycycline post-exposure prophylaxis for STI prevention among cisgender women. Chicago, IL: STI & HIV 2023 World Congress; 2023. Presented at.
7. Kirby Institute. Impact of the daily doxycycline pre-exposure prophylaxis (PrEP) on the incidence of syphilis, gonorrhoea and Chlamydia. clinicaltrials.gov; 2022. https://clinicaltrials.gov/study/NCT03709459.
8. CTN 329: Doxycycline Intervention for bacterial STI ChemoprOphylaxis (DISCO) | Prevention (PREV). CIHR Canadian HIV Trials Network. https://www.hivnet.ubc.ca/study/ctn-329-doxycycline-intervention-for-bacterial-sti-chemoprophylaxis-disco/.
9. CTN 313: The DaDHS Trial | Prevention (PREV). CIHR Canadian HIV Trials Network. https://www.hivnet.ubc.ca/study/ctn-313-the-dadhs-trial/.
10. Mylan Pharmaceuticals, Inc. Doxycycline Package Insert; 2016.
11. US Food & Drug Administration. Doxycycline Use by Pregnant and Lactating Women. https://www.fda.gov/drugs/bioterrorism-and-drug-preparedness/doxycycline-use-pregnant-and-lactating-women.
12. Vijay A, Valdes AM. Role of the gut microbiome in chronic diseases: a narrative review. Eur J Clin Nutr 2022;76(4):489–501.
13. Reichert E, Yaesoubi R, Rönn M, et al. Resistance-minimizing strategies for introducing a novel antibiotic for gonorrhea treatment: a mathematical modeling study. NY: Cold Spring Harbor; 2023.
14. Public Health - Seattle & King County HIV/STI/Hep C Program. Guidelines: Doxycycline Post-Exposure Prophylaxis (Doxy-PEP) to Prevent Bacterial STIs in Men who Have Sex with Men (MSM) and Transgender Persons who Have Sex with Men. Published online June 2023. https://kingcounty.gov/depts/health/communicable-diseases/hiv-std.aspx.
15. California Department of Public Health. Doxycycline Post-Exposure Prophylaxis (doxy-PEP) for the Prevention of Bacterial Sexually Transmitted Infections (STIs). Published online April 28, 2023. https://www.cdph.ca.gov/Programs/CID/DCDC/CDPH%20Document%20Library/CDPH-Doxy-PEP-Recommendations-for-Prevention-of-STIs.pdf.
16. Wiesenfeld HC, Lowry DL, Heine RP, et al. Self-collection of vaginal swabs for the detection of Chlamydia, gonorrhea, and trichomoniasis: opportunity to encourage sexually transmitted disease testing among adolescents. Sex Transm Dis 2001; 28(6):321–5.
17. van der Helm JJ, Hoebe CJPA, van Rooijen MS, et al. High Performance and Acceptability of Self-Collected Rectal Swabs for Diagnosis of Chlamydia trachomatis and Neisseria gonorrhoeae in Men Who Have Sex With Men and Women. Sex Transm Dis 2009;36(8):493–7.
18. Lunny C, Taylor D, Hoang L, et al. Self-Collected versus Clinician-Collected Sampling for Chlamydia and Gonorrhea Screening: A Systemic Review and Meta-Analysis. PLoS One 2015;10(7):e0132776.
19. Cantor A, Dana T, Griffin JC, et al. Screening for Chlamydial and Gonococcal Infections: A Systematic Review Update for the U.S. Preventive Services Task Force [Internet]. Rockville, MD: Agency for Healthcare Research and Quality (US); 2021.

20. Dangerfield DT, Farley JE, Holden J, et al. Acceptability of self-collecting oropharyngeal swabs for sexually transmissible infection testing among men and women. Sex Health 2019;16(3):296–8.
21. Kahn M, Van Der Pol B. Advances in Diagnostics of Sexually Transmitted Infections. Infect Dis Clin North Am 2023;37(2):381–403.
22. Van Der Pol B, Williams JA, Taylor SN, et al. Detection of Trichomonas vaginalis DNA by Use of Self-Obtained Vaginal Swabs with the BD ProbeTec Q ^{x} Assay on the BD Viper System. In: Gilligan PH, editor. J Clin Microbiol 2014;52(3):885–9.
23. Ogale Y, Yeh PT, Kennedy CE, et al. Self-collection of samples as an additional approach to deliver testing services for sexually transmitted infections: a systematic review and meta-analysis. BMJ Glob Health 2019;4(2).
24. Aptima Combo 2 Assay for CT/NG Package Insert | Hologic.
25. Barbee LA, Tat S, Dhanireddy S, et al. Implementation and Operational Research: Effectiveness and Patient Acceptability of a Sexually Transmitted Infection Self-Testing Program in an HIV Care Setting. J Acquir Immune Defic Syndr 1999 2016;72(2):e26–31.
26. Fajardo-Bernal L, Aponte-Gonzalez J, Vigil P, et al. Home-based versus clinic-based specimen collection in the management of Chlamydia trachomatis and Neisseria gonorrhoeae infections. Cochrane Database Syst Rev 2015;2015(9): CD011317.
27. Gaydos CA. Let's Take A "Selfie": Self-Collected Samples for Sexually Transmitted Infections. Sex Transm Dis 2018;45(4):278.
28. Gaydos CA, Van Der Pol B, Jett-Goheen M, et al. Performance of the Cepheid CT/NG Xpert Rapid PCR Test for Detection of Chlamydia trachomatis and Neisseria gonorrhoeae. J Clin Microbiol 2013;51(6):1666–72.
29. Adamson PC, Loeffelholz MJ, Klausner JD. Point-of-Care Testing for Sexually Transmitted Infections: A Review of Recent Developments. Arch Pathol Lab Med 2020;144(11):1344–51.
30. Gaydos CA, Manabe YC, Melendez JH. A Narrative Review of Where We Are With Point-of-Care Sexually Transmitted Infection Testing in the United States. Sex Transm Dis 2021;48(8S):S71–7.
31. Gaydos CA, Ako MC, Lewis M, et al. Use of a Rapid Diagnostic for Chlamydia trachomatis and Neisseria gonorrhoeae for Women in the Emergency Department Can Improve Clinical Management: Report of a Randomized Clinical Trial. Ann Emerg Med 2019;74(1):36–44.
32. May L, Ware CE, Jordan JA, et al. A Randomized Controlled Trial Comparing the Treatment of Patients Tested for Chlamydia and Gonorrhea After a Rapid Polymerase Chain Reaction Test Versus Standard of Care Testing. Sex Transm Dis 2016;43(5):290–5.
33. Wingrove I, McOwan A, Nwokolo N, et al. Diagnostics within the clinic to test for gonorrhoea and chlamydia reduces the time to treatment: a service evaluation. Sex Transm Infect 2014;90(6):474.
34. Shannon CL, Keizur EM, Fehrenbacher A, et al. Sexually Transmitted Infection Positivity Among Adolescents With or at High-Risk for Human Immunodeficiency Virus Infection in Los Angeles and New Orleans. Sex Transm Dis 2019;46(11): 737–42.
35. Keizur EM, Goldbeck C, Vavala G, et al. Safety and Effectiveness of Same-Day Chlamydia trachomatis and Neisseria gonorrhoeae Screening and Treatment Among Gay, Bisexual, Transgender, and Homeless Youth in Los Angeles, California, and New Orleans, Louisiana. Sex Transm Dis 2020;47(1):19–23.

36. Centers for Disease Control and Prevention. Sexually transmitted disease surveillance 2021. Atlanta, GA: US Dept of Health and Human Services; 2023.
37. Gliddon HD, Peeling RW, Kamb ML, et al. A systematic review and meta-analysis of studies evaluating the performance and operational characteristics of dual point-of-care tests for HIV and syphilis. Sex Transm Infect 2017;93(S4):S3–15.
38. Pham MD, Ong JJ, Anderson DA, et al. Point-of-Care Diagnostics for Diagnosis of Active Syphilis Infection: Needs, Challenges and the Way Forward. Int J Environ Res Publ Health 2022;19(13):8172.
39. Sadiq ST, Mazzaferri F, Unemo M. Rapid accurate point-of-care tests combining diagnostics and antimicrobial resistance prediction for Neisseria gonorrhoeae and Mycoplasma genitalium. Sex Transm Infect 2017;93(S4):S65–8.
40. Trick AY, Melendez JH, Chen FE, et al. A portable magnetofluidic platform for detecting sexually transmitted infections and antimicrobial susceptibility. Sci Transl Med 2021;13(593):eabf6356.
41. Craig AP, Gray RT, Edwards JL, et al. The potential impact of vaccination on the prevalence of gonorrhea. Vaccine 2015;33(36):4520–5.
42. Petousis-Harris H, Radcliff FJ. Exploitation of Neisseria meningitidis Group B OMV Vaccines Against N. gonorrhoeae to Inform the Development and Deployment of Effective Gonorrhea Vaccines. Front Immunol 2019;10:683.
43. Leduc I, Connolly KL, Begum A, et al. The serogroup B meningococcal outer membrane vesicle-based vaccine 4CMenB induces cross-species protection against Neisseria gonorrhoeae. PLoS Pathog 2020;16(12):e1008602.
44. Semchenko EA, Tan A, Borrow R, et al. The Serogroup B Meningococcal Vaccine Bexsero Elicits Antibodies to Neisseria gonorrhoeae. Clin Infect Dis Off Publ Infect Dis Soc Am 2019;69(7):1101–11.
45. Whelan J, Kløvstad H, Haugen IL, et al. Ecologic Study of Meningococcal B Vaccine and Neisseria gonorrhoeae Infection, Norway. Emerg Infect Dis 2016;22(6): 1137–9.
46. Bruxvoort KJ, Lewnard JA, Chen LH, et al. Prevention of Neisseria gonorrhoeae With Meningococcal B Vaccine: A Matched Cohort Study in Southern California. Clin Infect Dis Off Publ Infect Dis Soc Am 2023;76(3):e1341–9.
47. Molina JM. Meningitis B vaccine for prevention of gonorrhoea: what is the evidence? Brisbane, Australia: IAS 2023; 2023. Presented at.
48. Thng C, Semchenko EA, Hughes I, et al. An open-label randomised controlled trial evaluating the efficacy of a meningococcal serogroup B (4CMenB) vaccine on Neisseria gonorrhoeae infection in gay and bisexual men: the MenGO study protocol. BMC Publ Health 2023;23(1):607.
49. Johnson B. GSK's gonorrhea vaccine receives fast-track designation to expedite clinical trials. Nat Med 2023;29(9):2146–7.
50. Miller JN. Immunity in experimental syphilis. VI. Successful vaccination of rabbits with Treponema pallidum, Nichols strain, attenuated by -irradiation. J Immunol Baltim Md 1950 1973;110(5):1206–15.
51. Ávila-Nieto C, Pedreño-López N, Mitjà O, et al. Syphilis vaccine: challenges, controversies and opportunities. Front Immunol 2023;14:1126170.
52. Haynes AM, Giacani L, Mayans MV, et al. Efficacy of linezolid on Treponema pallidum, the syphilis agent: A preclinical study. EBioMedicine 2021;65:103281.
53. Edmondson DG, Hu B, Norris SJ. Long-Term In Vitro Culture of the Syphilis Spirochete Treponema pallidum subsp. pallidum. mBio 2018;9(3):e1218.
54. Lieberman NAP, Armstrong TD, Chung B, et al. High-throughput nanopore sequencing of Treponema pallidum tandem repeat genes arp and tp0470 reveals

clade-specific patterns and recapitulates global whole genome phylogeny. Front Microbiol 2022;13:1007056.
55. Lukehart SA, Molini B, Gomez A, et al. Immunization with a tri-antigen syphilis vaccine significantly attenuates chancre development, reduces bacterial load, and inhibits dissemination of Treponema pallidum. Vaccine 2022;40(52):7676–92.
56. Abraham S, Juel HB, Bang P, et al. Safety and immunogenicity of the chlamydia vaccine candidate CTH522 adjuvanted with CAF01 liposomes or aluminium hydroxide: a first-in-human, randomised, double-blind, placebo-controlled, phase 1 trial. Lancet Infect Dis 2019;19(10):1091–100.
57. Bergman H, Buckley BS, Villanueva G, et al. Comparison of different human papillomavirus (HPV) vaccine types and dose schedules for prevention of HPV-related disease in females and males. Cochrane Database Syst Rev 2019; 2019(11):CD013479.
58. Oshman LD, Davis AM. Human Papillomavirus Vaccination for Adults: Updated Recommendations of the Advisory Committee on Immunization Practices (ACIP). JAMA 2020;323(5):468–9.
59. Prudden HJ, Achilles SL, Schocken C, et al. Understanding the public health value and defining preferred product characteristics for therapeutic human papillomavirus (HPV) vaccines: World Health Organization consultations, October 2021-March 2022. Vaccine 2022;40(41):5843–55.
60. World Health Organization. Strategic advisory group of experts on immunization. Geneva, Switzerland: SAGE; 2022.
61. World Health Organization. Human papillomavirus vaccines. Geneva, Switzerland: WHO position paper; 2022.
62. Porras C, Sampson JN, Herrero R, et al. Rationale and design of a double-blind randomized non-inferiority clinical trial to evaluate one or two doses of vaccine against human papillomavirus including an epidemiologic survey to estimate vaccine efficacy: The Costa Rica ESCUDDO trial. Vaccine 2022;40(1):76–88.
63. Shannon CL, Bristow C, Hoff N, et al. Acceptability and Feasibility of Rapid Chlamydial, Gonococcal, and Trichomonal Screening and Treatment in Pregnant Women in 6 Low- to Middle-Income Countries. Sex Transm Dis 2018;45(10):673–6.
64. Fuller SS, Clarke E, Harding-Esch EM. Molecular chlamydia and gonorrhoea point of care tests implemented into routine practice: Systematic review and value proposition development. PLoS One 2021;16(11):e0259593.
65. Van Der Pol B, Taylor SN, Mena L, et al. Evaluation of the Performance of a Point-of-Care Test for Chlamydia and Gonorrhea. JAMA Netw Open 2020;3(5):e204819.
66. Widdice LE, Hsieh YH, Silver B, et al. Performance of the Atlas Genetics Rapid Test for Chlamydia trachomatis and Women's Attitudes Toward Point-Of-Care Testing. Sex Transm Dis 2018;45(11):723–7.
67. Van Der Pol B, Gaydos CA. A profile of the binx health io® molecular point-of-care test for chlamydia and gonorrhea in women and men. Expert Rev Mol Diagn 2021;21(9):861–8.
68. Morris SR, Bristow CC, Wierzbicki MR, et al. Performance of a single-use, rapid, point-of-care PCR device for the detection of Neisseria gonorrhoeae, Chlamydia trachomatis, and Trichomonas vaginalis: a cross-sectional study. Lancet Infect Dis 2021;21(5):668–76.
69. Dawkins M, Bishop L, Walker P, et al. Clinical Integration of a Highly Accurate Polymerase Chain Reaction Point-of-Care Test Can Inform Immediate Treatment Decisions for Chlamydia, Gonorrhea, and Trichomonas. Sex Transm Dis 2022; 49(4):262–7.

70. Schwebke JR, Gaydos CA, Davis T, et al. Clinical Evaluation of the Cepheid Xpert TV Assay for Detection of Trichomonas vaginalis with Prospectively Collected Specimens from Men and Women. J Clin Microbiol 2018;56(2):e1117.
71. Gaydos CA, Schwebke J, Dombrowski J, et al. Clinical performance of the Solana® Point-of-Care Trichomonas Assay from clinician-collected vaginal swabs and urine specimens from symptomatic and asymptomatic women. Expert Rev Mol Diagn 2017;17(3):303–6.
72. Gaydos CA, Klausner JD, Pai NP, et al. Rapid and point-of-care tests for the diagnosis of Trichomonas vaginalis in women and men. Sex Transm Infect 2017; 93(S4):S31–5.

Moving?

Make sure your subscription moves with you!

To notify us of your new address, find your **Clinics Account Number** (located on your mailing label above your name), and contact customer service at:

Email: journalscustomerservice-usa@elsevier.com

800-654-2452 **(subscribers in the U.S. & Canada)**
314-447-8871 **(subscribers outside of the U.S. & Canada)**

Fax number: 314-447-8029

Elsevier Health Sciences Division
Subscription Customer Service
3251 Riverport Lane
Maryland Heights, MO 63043

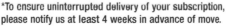

*To ensure uninterrupted delivery of your subscription, please notify us at least 4 weeks in advance of move.

ELSEVIER

Printed and bound by CPI Group (UK) Ltd, Croydon, CR0 4YY
03/10/2024
01040467-0020